AF223886

Instructions for using AR

LET AUGMENTED REALITY CHANGE HOW YOU READ A BOOK

With your smartphone, iPad or tablet you can use the **Hasmark AR** app to invoke the augmented reality experience to literally read outside the book.

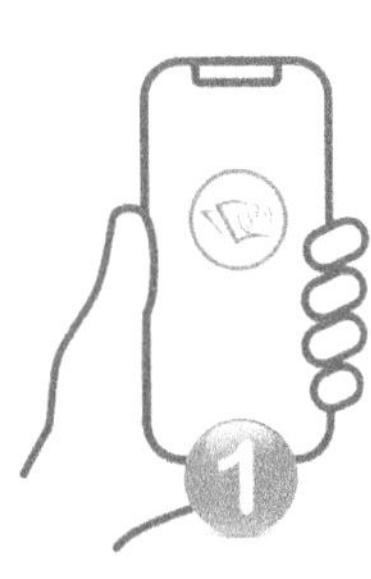

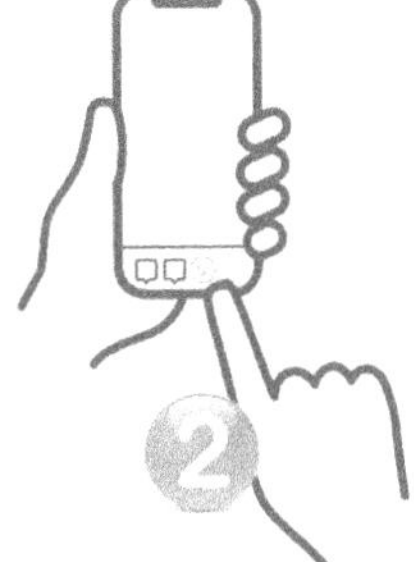

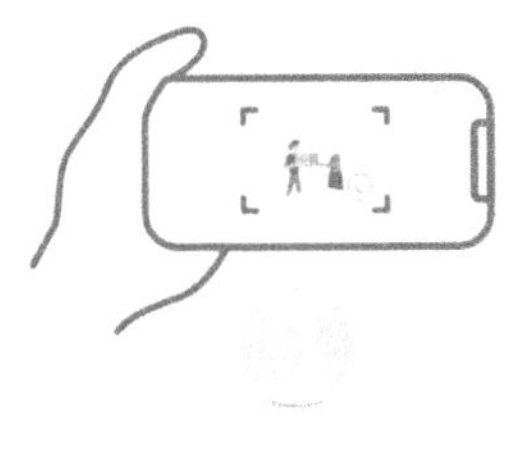

1. Download the **Hasmark app** from the **Apple App Store** or **Google Play**

2. Open and select the  (vue) option

3. Point your lens at the full image with the and enjoy the augmented reality experience.

Go ahead and try it right now with the Hasmark Publishing International logo.

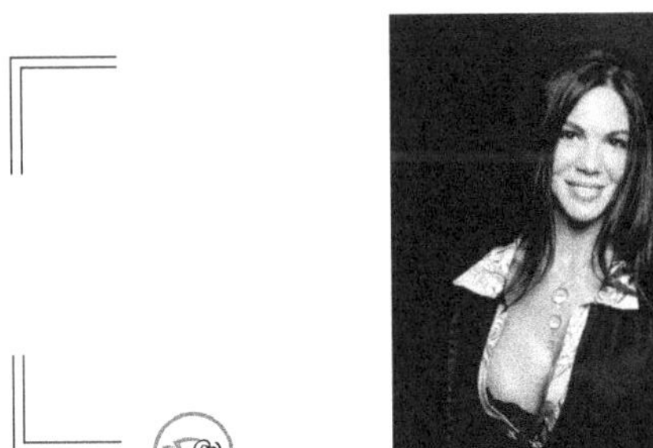

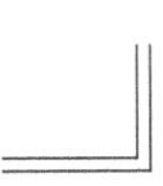

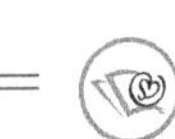

ENDORSEMENTS

Nerves of Steele is a bare knuckled, literary "selfie" of a woman who refused to be swept along by dysfunctional relationships and domestic tedium, myopically working her way up to become a successful businesswoman, courageous Mother, and one of social media's most desirable women. Most people are defined by their trials and traumas but Linda Steele (an apt moniker for such a strong person) would not succumb. Rather, she marshalled (and marketed) her unique skills and achieved personal and professional success on her own terms. Something so few of us are ever able to do.

—**William Ostrander**, Actor and
Political Activist

The saying "Don't Judge a book by its cover" could never be truer than the new book ***Nerves of Steele***. I remember five years ago seeing photos of Linda Steele online and watching a few of her YouTube videos. At that time, I assumed that she was someone who had it all, who had an easy road to reaching her achievements. But after reading her book, I discovered that my assumption was not accurate at all. ***Nerves of Steele*** is Elite Fitness Trainer/Gym Owner/Figure Model/Actress Linda Steele's memoir about overcoming an abusive stepfather, negligent husband, controlling boyfriend and a whirlwind of jet setting romances to build her brand to what it is today. Back in 2017, I reached out to Linda to try to cast her as an actress in my award-winning psychological suspense-thriller *Terry R. Wickham's Double Vision*. At that time, she turned me down telling me that she was not an actress and didn't have time to become one. Reading what was going on in her life during that time certainly illuminated me to why she declined. Three years later in February 2021, I pitched the lead role of "Officer Rachel Langer" to Linda in my to-be-filmed next year supernatural suspense feature film *Terry R. Wickham's Anomaly* and this time she accepted. We shot a Teaser Trailer together for investors in February 2022 in New Jersey. Having worked with Linda in person, I got to know of her honest tender heart and commitment to whatever it is she tackles. You too can have the chance to learn why Linda Steele's tumultuous story is much more than meets the eye.

—**Terry R. Wickham**, Writer/Producer/Director,
Terry R. Wickham's Anomaly/Devil's Five/
Terry R. Wickham's Double Vision

This book is an amazing story and very inspirational. It shows the reader how to overcome adversity and setbacks, yet stay true to your ideals. A major achievement!

—**Stewart St Clair**, UK HEALTH Radio

Fitness icon Linda Steele's book *Nerves of Steele* is an inspirational triumph of spirit and positivity energy. This book will resonate with everyone who reads it. It's real and raw, revealing pain and heartache, but showing strength and determination to overcome and succeed. Linda details childhood trauma and how it carries over into adulthood, and how the experience made her who she is today: a mother, iconic fitness personality and successful businesswoman. I highly recommend it as a must read!!

—**Jimmy Star,** #1 Webshow in The World,
www.jimmystarsworld.com

Nerves of Steele is a harrowing account of the life of world-renowned fitness personality Linda Steele. The detailed depth she shares with the world is a huge inspiration to everyone on the planet. Childhood abuse, bad relationships, creating your identity while raising children and building a business are all incredible stories, turning tragedy into personal triumph. Linda Steele should be named the 8th wonder of the world, thanks so much for sharing your story!!!

—**Ron Russell**, The Jimmy Star and Ron Russell Show,
#1 Webshow in The World

Nerves of Steele is a testament to what one person can do in the face of adversity, abuse, and insecurities to follow their dreams. *Nerves of Steele* is a gripping achievement to the perseverance and determination of an individual who went through so much, and yet was able to find her footing in an age of unbelievable obstacles. It a profoundly down to earth and understandably emotional from the beginning to end. It showcases a path of unbelievable trauma that morphs into astonishing wisdom and realistic hope. *Nerves of Steele* is for those who continuously go through dark nights and can't see their way clear: this book will show a lit path to a brighter and better tomorrow.

—**Monteque Pope-Le Beau,** Founder of Dreamweaverarts
organization, Artist, Poet, Playwright,
The Art Of Monteque, Art is Life and Life is Art,
http:/www.theartofmonteque.com

Nerves of Steele gets the 4E's of Movie Reviews and More: Its Engrossing, Educational, Entertaining and Emotional.

—**Brian Sebastian,** Movie Reviews and More,
Dreamweaver Arts

Linda Steele and I became friends a couple years ago. Our friendship was immediate mostly because we thought alike. She is the most motivated person I have ever met. And just like Linda, I NEVER played the victim. Her book, *Nerves of Steele*, is a testament to Linda's character and a must read!

—**Tim Tyrrell,** Friend & 7 Year NFL Player,
Atlanta Falcons 1984 -1986, LA Rams 1986 – 1988,
Buffalo Bills 1989, Pittsburgh Steelers 1989 - 1990

Trying to encapsulate Linda Steele in a few short sentences is utterly impossible, because how does one define a real-life superhero? It is often said that nothing worth doing comes easy and Linda's life story reflects this over and over again. She could have folded and embraced "easy" literally dozens of times before she reached voting age. Instead, Linda persisted. Linda fought. Linda persevered. Now, Linda is sharing her story of inspiration and resilience to add to the legions of lives she has transformed as one of the nation's top personal trainers.

—**Ryan McCrary**, PR, Communications &
Content Professional Worldwide

Nerves of Steele is a very strong story that inspires others to never give up hope. Linda's journey will show you that you are not alone, and everything in life happens for a reason.

—**Athena Vas,** Actor/Writer,
Warner Bros. The Bachelor Winner

Nerves of Steele

A MEMOIR

LINDA STEELE

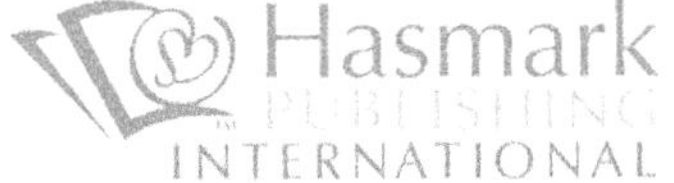

Published by
Hasmark Publishing International
www.hasmarkpublishing.com

Copyright © 2023 Linda Steele
First Edition

No part of this book may be reproduced or transmitted in any form or by any means, electronic or mechanical, including photocopying, recording or by any information storage and retrieval system, without written permission from the author, except for the inclusion of brief quotations in a review.

Disclaimer

This book is designed to provide information and motivation to our readers. It is sold with the understanding that the publisher is not engaged to render any type of psychological, legal, or any other kind of professional advice. The content of this book is the sole expression and opinion of its author, and not necessarily that of the publisher. No warranties or guarantees are expressed or implied by the publisher's choice to include any of the content in this volume. Neither the publisher nor the individual author(s) shall be liable for any physical, psychological, emotional, financial, or commercial damages, including, but not limited to, special, incidental, consequential or other damages. Our views and rights are the same: You are responsible for your own choices, actions, and results.

Permission should be addressed in writing to Linda Steele at Linda@ LindaSteeleWellness.com

Editor: Deanna Novak deanna@thewritejourneys.com
Cover Design: Anne Karklins anne@hasmarkpublishing.com
Interior Layout: Amit Dey amit@hasmarkpublishing.com

ISBN 13: 978-1-77482-124-4
ISBN 10: 1774821249

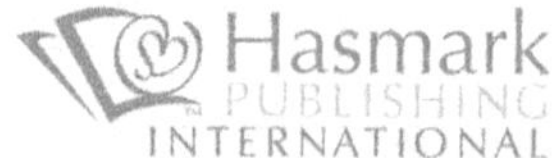

DEDICATION

I dedicate this book to my beautiful daughters. There are not enough words to describe the love I have for each of you. Continue to move mountains and never, ever let anything stand in your way.

I dedicate this book to my mom. I love you and I'm so grateful you're still with me to share this book as a lesson to the world.

I dedicate this book to my dad. I wish nothing more than to still have you by my side.

TABLE OF CONTENTS

ACKNOWLEDGMENTS

I could not complete this book without thanking the people who have supported me along my journey. Thank you …

To my daughters. I've been thanking God for the opportunity to be your mom every day since I knew I was pregnant. And just like any mom, there are things I wish I could have done better, but I hope you learned some lessons out of the mistakes I've made. My primary job, and the best gift I could give you, was to prepare you for life. You can take my experiences and decide how you want to live based on how things turned out for me, and for us. Each one of you has taught me something different in life, as well. I'm watching in awe as you conduct your lives in such a way that I wished I had done sooner. I cherish every minute we spend together with all the laughs, the tears, and everything in between. I'm so proud of the women you've become.

To my mom. It wasn't until I became an adult that I understood the decisions you made in your life. You did what you had to do for survival, and you did what was right at the time. I have not walked a mile in your stilettos, but I have walked a mile in my own, and I can easily draw a parallel to your life. You taught me how to adapt and you taught me how to push back, even if what you could gain from it was temporary. Your unconditional love and support have been what has driven me. I knew that I "could" because you told me, "You can."

To my dad. It's because of you that I expect my car doors to be opened, my coat to be put on, my chair to be pulled out, and for a man to walk streetside. You weren't around to see me in a healthy relationship. You tried to guide me in certain lessons, but I had to learn myself … and in my own time. I miss you terribly, every day of my life, but I appreciate what I was able to learn from you more than I can say.

To my Sissy. The amount of unconditional love you have given me from the minute I was born is second to none. You would stand in front of a freight train for me, no questions asked. Your passion, temperament, and spirit are what everyone around you envies most. I've never met a more loyal person in my life, and I thank God every day that you are on my side. I love you.

To Touchdown. You are my best friend and you taught me how to let someone love me. I've been knocked down more times than I can count, but somehow, at my most vulnerable moments, you make me feel like I'm still in control. You have the answers to questions I'm unclear about and encourage me to do what I love without fear, anxiety, doubt, or worry. I love you for that! Thank you for sharing me with the world.

To my family. You watched me grow through my transition to who I am today. No one likes change, but you all accepted me and trusted the process for me to reach my end goal. I love all of you for that, but most of all, I love all of you for the fond memories that I hold deep in my heart. I am so fortunate to have the closeness that I have with each one of you.

To my clients. Whether you have been with me for one month or eighteen years, you have seen firsthand what writing this book took out of me. Many of you have been with me on both my best and worst days, and you always stuck by my side. You are the reason I get excited to go to work each morning. I don't think anyone has a better job in the world than I do, and I am thankful for it every day.

To all my lifelong friends. You've witnessed everything in this book firsthand and you never stopped loving me and believing in me. Thank you for being there for me.

To Rick. I'll never forget how you were there when I was at my weakest. You were not going to let me fail, and you did everything in your power to let my brand go on without skipping a beat. You picked me up, helped me make decisions, and taught me about engaging with my fans. You encouraged and supported me always. I know there were days you felt like you were herding ducklings while working with me, yet you always managed to keep me on track.

To Ryan. What can I possibly say to express the gratitude for everything you've done over the years? You not only supported me, but you made me feel bigger and better than I ever felt before. You truly made me feel like a superhero on days that I just wanted to crumble. You made me laugh when I wanted to cry. You've been in my life a long time, and I will never forget how you helped me organize my thoughts for this book.

To Jim. You believed in me from the very beginning. You supported me in so many ways and always had great timing to help me find ways to advance myself, no matter what the cost.

To "Pinched." You appreciated me in many ways, and I hope you know how much I've appreciated you, as well. I could not have completed this book adventure without your support, your belief in me, and your encouragement. The work ethic that we share is our special bond. The time we spend bouncing ideas off each other has really helped us both understand the day-to-day in business and in life, and how to balance it all.

To Brian Sebastian. Meeting you was the link between promoting my brand and writing this book. You have introduced me to the most unique and interesting people from L.A. to Nashville, and places in between. You have pushed me to my limits and encouraged me to follow through on things that I never thought I would.

To Stuart Pearce. My time cohosting with you on the UK health radio was the start of me deciding what I wanted my future to look like. I love to teach, and that's what I do, but getting my voice out there to tens of thousands of people at a time is what I love even more. Thank you for that opportunity. That trip to London in 2020 was a game changer for me. You introduced me to all the right people who made me believe in myself enough to start this book.

To AJ Joshi. I will never forget the phone calls when you allowed me to be vulnerable, even though all you had known was my tough side. You were one of the people who reminded me that there was nothing I couldn't do with my life. You may not know it, but you gave me the courage to pick myself up and try when I didn't want to.

To my photographers. You were so patient with me. I appreciate you all for such different reasons, but mostly for reminding me who I was. You were at the very beginning of me getting my groove back. I will never forget the role each one of you has played in my life. Through patience, understanding, and emotional support, you became more than my photographers—you became my friends.

To Deanna Novak from The Write Journeys. You helped make my words even more powerful and my story have a life of its own. I cannot thank you enough.

To Banafsheh Akhlaghi, Akhlaghi Law. Your guidance throughout this entire process was more hands on than I could have ever expected. I appreciate how thorough and detailed you were. Thank you.

To the entire Hasmark team. From the front cover design to the marketing guidance I received. I cannot imagine a better team behind me in making this idea come to life. I appreciate every detail that went into each decision made.

PREFACE

Writing this book has been on my list of things to do for several years, but because I was in such a good place, I put it off. When confronting childhood trauma, there is a tendency to use "selective amnesia" as a coping mechanism. As we know, the brain does its best to protect itself, much like any other body part that is injured. Still, once I got started, I found myself recalling things I had long since "forgotten."

Confronting the past is difficult. It takes courage, in and of itself, but coming to terms with it is essential to healing. For years, I couldn't help but feel sorry for myself for the things I had to deal with daily at such a young age. But as they say, our pasts—the good, the bad, and the ugly—make us who we are today. And that's amazing if you like yourself today, but that does not make it any easier to relive it, and then, to write about it in detail.

This book forced me to remember things I deliberately chose to forget—not just in my childhood, but through my adult years, as well. It's safe to say, I've had my fair share of heartache. But I know now that growing up in a household that replaced encouragement with mental and verbal abuse, comforting hugs with inappropriate touching, happy marriages with divorces, thriving teens with teen pregnancies, and family dinners with drugs and alcohol abuse actually shaped me into the strong, determined, courageous woman I am today. The woman who will not tolerate anything less than what I deserve.

I know exactly how this is going to go. I will get through the painstaking process of writing it and I will never read it again. But knowing I had the courage to fully reflect on the traumas, the lows, the lowers, and some exceptional triumphs through it all is really enough for me. I am not the only one to experience childhood trauma that shaped the parameters and intricacies of later relationships. I fully understand that. My hope is that my story can serve as a raw, unfiltered example that even through the darkest times, it is possible to rise above them. What we don't realize when we're going through it is that each challenge, each heartache, each tear is building us up stronger than ever before so that we can conquer whatever is thrown our way next.

This book may parallel your life in many ways. I hope it will provide some comfort in showing you that you are not alone, but not in a "pity party" way. Instead, I want you to realize that no matter what is thrown your way, no matter how shitty the circumstances appear, you are strong enough not only to take it, but to use it as fuel to propel you higher than you ever imagined. I want to empower you until you can learn to empower yourself even more.

What follows is not a fairytale. This is a true account of my life from start to finish. The phrase, "That which does not kill me makes me stronger" applies to many passages throughout my life. This is not to say that there have not been many highlights and unbelievable happiness and joy along the way. This is not to say I am not grateful for all of them—because I am. What it is to say is that I am living proof that you can be knocked down more times than you care to count and continue on to be successful, happy, and at peace.

My hope is that every person reading this can use it as a tool to inspire them to be better. To do better. To make better decisions. To convert negative energy into fuel for positive change. Make no mistake, none of the above is easy. The best things in life never, ever are.

PROLOGUE

Dispatch: "911, What's your emergency?"

Me: "My stepfather just hit my mommy."

Dispatch: "Okay. Did you see him hit her?"

Me: "No, I heard it. And I heard her fall, and scream like she was hurt, and I heard him strangling her. She was trying to scream."

Dispatch: "Is she ok?"

Me, more hysterical: "I don't know. I don't hear anything now."

Dispatch: "Okay, we are sending someone right away."

I was the only child home that night. I was alone in my bedroom. And I was scared to death … for my mom … and for me.

But I was brave. I've always been brave …

Chapter 1

IN THE BEGINNING

My parents divorced when I was two years old. I am not alone—many parents get divorced. Yet I am one of the very few people I know who does not blame any of my life's mishaps on that often life-altering event in a child's life. In fact, I am incredibly appreciative that they made the split when I was young, so I didn't have to adapt to any of the big changes other kids have to adjust to—holiday time, every other weekend visits, or any of the other shit that goes along with being a child with divorced parents. All I ever knew was that every Christmas Eve was with my mom and her family, and every Christmas Day was with my dad and his. And I loved spending time with each. Those earliest celebrations with each side of my family are some of my favorite childhood memories.

One similarity they had was that they both put great emphasis on having a close relationship with family. I have two older sisters. My middle sister and I never really got along. Through most of my interactions with her, I felt as if she was picking on me—even to the point of bullying. My relationship with my oldest sister, was the complete opposite. I always felt very loved and extremely protected by her. I loved any time I was with her. She had a way of calming me and making me feel special.

All of my cousins and I grew up together, seeing each other on weekends and spending family vacations together. My mom and I would travel once a month or so to Ludington, Michigan to see her parents. But it was never just them—there were aunts and uncles and always, my cousins. I have thirteen cousins between both sides of the family, and we were all born within ten years of each other. So, at different times, our lives were at vastly different stages. Still, our times together were always memorable.

One cousin taught me how to drive, another cousin invited me on a cruise with her for her senior class trip. I have special memories with each of my cousins that I treasure to this day. Some of us lived near each other and attended schools in the same district. We shared friends and sporting events. Even as adults, when most of these childhood relationships strain, we have managed to stay close.

Seven years after her divorce to my dad, my mother remarried. I knew our life was going to be different combining our families, but I had no idea how different. It was much more than moving from Chicago to Wheeling, after my mom and stepfather were married. When it was just me and my mom, we had fun together. She would take me shopping or to Kiddie-Land. Sometimes, we would just go for a ride in the car. And, of course, our trips to Ludington to see the family were always great.

Suddenly though, I became the youngest of eight children in our new mixed family. Five of them were my new stepbrothers, the other two were my sisters. While some of them were older and already out of the house, there were never less than four or five children living at home those first few years.

Growing up in this household, the irony was not lost on me that there were two television shows (*Eight is Enough* and *The Brady Bunch*) championing the triumph of combined families. Each episode had a crisis involving something as simple as a shattered vase or someone being caught smoking. And all issues were resolved in thirty minutes, tied up with a pretty pink bow, and fueled by a studio laugh track.

We definitely were not *The Brady Bunch*. To the best of my knowledge, on that show, Mike never mentally abused Carol or the step kids. The boys did not torment and mentally and, at times, physically, abuse their stepsisters to delight their father. Marcia did not get pregnant at sixteen. Jan did not have a nasty, consuming drug habit. Peter did not have sex in the house with Jan. It wasn't quite the same.

Despite the shows, growing up in my household seemed "normal" since it was the only reality I knew. But looking back now, I realize it was anything but normal—it was pure and utter chaos. My siblings would come and go due to marriages and divorces, teen pregnancies and babies out of wedlock, drug and alcohol abuse, and any other trauma you can imagine. Nothing surprised my mom and stepfather after a while, but these things did cause quite a bit of strain on the entire household. Somehow, they managed to hold their marriage together, despite my prayers that they wouldn't.

Don't get me wrong—I loved my stepfather when they first got together, but it wasn't long before I grew to hate him. When I met him, he seemed very kind and patient. My first recollection of him was when I was about three years old. He held me in his arms as we snuck carrots out of the soup that my mom had just made. He was being silly and sneaky, and my mom was playing mad that we were eating all the carrots out of the soup! It's actually one of the fondest memories I have of him.

We were close back then. If he was around, I was always sitting on his lap. If he had to run to the store, I'd tag along. While we would sit at the kitchen table waiting for my mom to finish making dinner, we'd play the game where he'd put his hand on mine, then, I'd put my hand on his, then he'd take his second hand and put it on top, I'd follow along. We would do this over and over until I'd start to giggle.

This playful relationship worked while they were dating, and we weren't together all the time. It ended quite abruptly after the families collided and moved under one roof. The silliness and playfulness morphed into something else entirely—something ugly and abhorrent. The turning point was the night I heard my stepfather hit my mother. The turning point was when I called the police on my stepfather.

Chapter 2

911 ... AND THEN SILENCE

I was about nine years old the night my entire universe shifted. It was dark out, almost bedtime, and I was playing with my Barbies in my bedroom. I overheard an argument between my mom and stepfather about my fourteen-year-old sister who was caught doing drugs again. Arguments were not unusual in our house, but I remember thinking, even at that very young age, that something was not right this time. I remember thinking I should maybe call the police. The yelling escalated much louder than usual and seemed more threatening somehow. Still, I was unsure. How was I to know? I hesitated ... and then I heard a slap. The next thing I heard was my mom hitting the floor and her screaming suddenly becoming muffled, as if she couldn't breathe. I ran out of my bedroom and passed their closed bedroom door, down the stairs, and into the kitchen, where I picked up the phone and dialed 911.

I went back up to my bedroom and shortly after, my mom came in my room. I was pacing, waiting for the police to arrive. I wasn't crying. I felt very brave in my decision. I asked her if she was ok, and she lifted her shirt to show me how when she fell, she hit her dresser first and it put a gash just below her ribcage. I told her I called the police, and she told me they heard. The doorbell rang, and I ran downstairs to answer the door, my mom trying to keep up behind me.

Two officers came into the foyer of the house and started asking my mom specifically what happened. I couldn't believe it as I heard her calmly tell them nothing was wrong. She denied that he did anything. I pointed out the visible mark she had on her side. The police asked me what I heard. I told them everything, even though my mom and stepfather were both looking at me like, "don't you even." I didn't care about their looks. I was going to tell the police the truth. The officers asked her if she wanted to file charges … she said no. My mom and stepfather said everything was fine, the police officers left—taking my life as I knew it with them.

I was so disappointed that my mom didn't stick up for herself. I felt like she abandoned me. Just left me hanging out there like some child who had too big of an imagination. I knew what I heard, and I knew right from wrong. She always taught me right from wrong. How could she miss this one? As an adult, I understand now that she was torn. Of course, she wanted to tell the police what happened. Of course, she wanted to stick by my side. But she was balancing those wants with the incredible fear of what would happen to her if she said or did anything other than what he wanted. She was worried about the physical pain she would endure and even where we would live. But, to me, at that moment in time, all I felt was isolation—it was them against me.

The police incident was never discussed again. Mom never treated me any differently, and even secretly told me I did the right thing. I appreciated that, but it still fell short of what I thought it would be. Yet there were other changes happening. This was when my stepfather stopped abusing my mom and started abusing me.

My stepfather stopped talking to me, acknowledging me, or even looking at me. He wouldn't say, "Hello," when I greeted him. Every time I accomplished something—whether I made the cheerleading squad or the volleyball team or the softball team or was elected to student council—my mom would tell him while we sat at the dinner table. And he'd say nothing—NOTHING—in return. It was as if she hadn't said a word, as if I didn't exist at all. He wouldn't acknowledge my birthdays, or my very presence … ever.

Initially, the way he treated me was very disappointing. But instead of letting it take me down, I had an "Aha moment"—at a very young age. I realized I would take the toxicity and use it as fuel to drive me forward. I remember saying in my head, "Fuck you, what do I need your applause for? You are a piece of shit."

For years, I tried to tell myself that maybe it was ok. Maybe it was even a good thing that he ignored me. But then I remember that I was not even ten years old at the time, and I had loved him very much. I wanted to be recognized. I wanted to be valued. I wanted to be loved, especially by the people I loved most. At that age, attention—whether positive or negative—is something you crave. Being completely ignored is incredibly cruel and damaging to a young person who is still developing and trying to figure out who they are.

Once, nearly five years after I had called the police, when I was about fourteen years old, I actually *thought* he was talking to me. We had been on a trip to Ludington to visit my grandparents and he happened to come with us this time. I had also brought my friend Jan (he never spoke to her either, but she was used to it by now, so she wasn't offended—maybe intimidated, but not offended.) I had met Jan soon after we moved to Wheeling. So, she had witnessed this absurd family dynamics in my household for years when she would come over to play. She, unfortunately, knew exactly what she was getting herself into by coming with us on this trip. Knowing neither of us could change how he treated us; we would just shake our heads and giggle behind his back at how ridiculous he looked bullying little girls.

At breakfast that day, I recall the four of us were sitting across the table from each other at McDonald's. Jan and I were both looking down at our food and eating, quiet, as always, when we were near him. Then, suddenly, we both heard him ask, "How are your pancakes?" After several seconds, I realized no one answered him, so I looked up thinking he might be talking to me. As it turned out, he was looking directly at Jan. I hit Jan on her leg to get her attention. She quickly looked up noticing that he was addressing her, and I thought she was going to choke on her pancakes. She stuttered a response, "Um, they're good." I'm pretty sure those were the only words he ever spoke to Jan. Needless to say, Jan and I had to hide the giggling in the backseat all the way home because we were in shock.

While I recall this incident with a smile on my face because it was not as isolated as usual, overall, the mental strain his actions put on me was unbearable. I became very sad, angry, resentful, and physically sick with a variety of symptoms. I had *debilitating* migraines and severe stomach pains, resulting in monthly, if not weekly, visits to the pediatrician. If he wasn't completely ignoring me, he would shake his head or roll his eyes with an utter look of disgust every time I caught his eye. It was slowly, but surely, destroying my young, impressionable spirit.

Chapter 3

HOUSE OF HORRORS

Often, what hurt me even more was that everyone saw how my step-father treated me and no one ever stood up for me. No one ever told him it was wrong to treat a young girl so cruelly. Not my mom. Not my siblings. No one. It was obvious and uncomfortable, all the time. And it was ignored by everyone until much later in life. My oldest sister was somewhat removed from the situation because she had too much of her own drama to deal with. She got pregnant at sixteen and moved out of the house. As you can imagine, I would have been her last concern, if I was any concern at all.

Mom would try in her own ways though. Her attempt at helping the situation was having us all be together more. I think she was thinking that maybe having all of us around at once would soften my stepfather. I think she hoped that maybe if we all got to know each other, we would start to like one another. I think deep down, most of us wanted the same thing, but it didn't change the fact that my stepfather appeared to play us against each other. It was no secret that he felt that his boys should be treated with superiority.

Unfortunately, my mom's attempts at bringing us together only tore us apart even more. This "family time" didn't instill any sense of mutual respect or admiration. Instead, it created the perfect platform for my stepbrothers to please their father. They must have known how he felt about me (everyone did), so they took every opportunity to tease me or ignore me completely in front of him. If I did have enough courage to speak (in my own home), all it would take was misusing a word or asking a question to be completely humiliated by one or all of them at once.

Much like you see in wildlife documentaries, the weakest in the herd are always the first to be targeted by predators. In my story, the role of the predator was played not only by my stepfather, but also by a cast of, what I considered, deplorables made up of my disgusting stepbrothers. And just like in those documentaries, I had to do whatever it took to survive.

Other times, I was just ignored, following their father's example, as if I didn't exist—as if I had no voice at all. I never imagined being ignored by everyone might have been the safest thing for me when faced with verbal, mental, and physical abuse. I am not going to try to figure out why they choose one method over another at different times because it does not matter how they mistreated me, the fact is that I felt bullied and abused in the place where I should have found the most comfort.

My stepbrothers had another ally besides my stepfather though. They had my sister. From what I remember feeling and what I've been told by other family members, she hated me since the day I was born. It was far beyond any sibling rivalry I have ever heard of. And now, she didn't have to mistreat me herself because she had others do it for her. It seemed as though she would instigate my stepbrothers and encourage them to treat me horribly. The more they made me cry, the more it would escalate. One of my stepbrothers, in particular, used her as reinforcement, like bullies do, as they verbally, mentally, and physically abused me. It would be nothing to them to give me a swift smack to the back of the head as they walked past me, for no reason at all. It wasn't a stretch to see why I was at doctor's appointments for ulcers and migraines for years.

When my spirit was beaten down, I would retreat to the safety and solitude of my bedroom. I would bury myself in homework or organizing my clothes or toys. What was so confusing to me, and the single reason why I just didn't hide within the confines of my room all the time was because *some* of the time, *some* of the boys were actually nice to me—as long as their dad wasn't around to see it. This is what kept me coming back for more. I thought, "maybe this time they will like me." I could only compare it to the game of golf … when you have a good drive, you're anxious to drive again. Yet, more often than not, I was disappointed.

There were things that went on in that household that I will not mention. And sometimes, I was hurt beyond words. I honestly cannot imagine what the fuck was going through their sick heads when grossly inappropriate actions were taking place. I have blocked the details as much as possible, but it was during this time that I realized I had to have my guard up and not trust any of them. I was disgusted and disappointed almost every day of my life for years.

In healthy family dynamics, brothers are supposed to look after and protect their younger siblings in general (little sisters, in particular). This simply did not exist. I don't think that I imagined that the bullying primarily went on when my stepfather was watching. One on one, they were usually pretty nice to me. The one I spent most of my time with was nice about 50% of the time, but he was hard to read and very hot and cold. I never knew when he was going to be great or awful, but it usually depended on if his dad was there. It wasn't until years later that I was able to see what they were doing. It seemed like they were showing off, trying to please him themselves. That was when they had the stage, and their dad was the audience. Sadly, his measure of worth for his children was how awful they could be.

I was a little girl. Some of them were grown men—grown men who should have protected me, not tormented me for sport. They ranged from six to eighteen years older than me. It is sickening that picking on a little girl made them feel good, regardless of who was watching. Imagine a 30-year-old picking on a preteen for someone else's approval. It's sad to think how badly they thought of themselves deep down to be so anxious for their father's praise.

While my stepbrothers had their allies, I had one too—my older sister. They say that it takes a bigger bully to conquer bullies, and she had no fear in that respect. She was the kind of sister who throughout my life would stop at nothing to protect me from anyone who was picking on me. She is the kind of woman who would bring a gun to a knife fight, so to speak. She was the closest to anyone who stood up for me with the abuse that went on in my home. The way she did that was to be a bigger bully to the boys, including my stepfather, than they were to me.

They always wondered why she had such a big chip on her shoulder when she came by for a family dinner. She would barely speak to any of the boys, and if they were being nice to me, and I was being nice back, she would remind me they were not good people. She was right. But as a little girl, I just remember constantly craving their approval, so if they were nice, I ate it up and was a sweetheart back. I didn't realize I was only leaving myself open for disappointment as they used that vulnerable time to tease me and make me feel stupid again.

Eventually, my other sister, the bully, was kicked out of the house and moved in with our dad. This took some of the tension out of the mix (my stepbrothers lost an instigator and ally), but the next several years of my life are still very foggy. I have no recollection of weekday family dinners, but I do know that my mom cooked dinner every night for the family. I am not sure if my brain blocked it out because it was so painful to relive the teasing and vicious arguments that usually occurred then.

What I remember most is eating quietly with my mom and stepfather, and occasionally, one of my stepbrothers. There would be very little conversation between them, and none that included me. My mom and stepfather would say a few words back and forth. She would always ask him about his day. He never asked her about hers. She would try to ask about my day, but he would make it very uncomfortable with pure looks of disgust every time I opened my mouth. So, I adapted. As much as I wanted to talk to my mom, I would give very short answers with hopes that she would turn the conversation back over to him, and I could just finish my dinner in peace and go back to my room.

I knew what a healthy family dynamic should look like and feel like. I saw bits and pieces of it in the homes of my aunts and uncles. I saw bits and pieces of it in my friend's homes. I thank God for the first friend I met when we moved to the suburbs, Gina. I spent a lot of time at her house and playing outside with her and other friends in the neighborhood. As I grew into a teen, I would spend hours at my friend's houses, Marlene's and Jan's, where I felt like their moms and dads were always trying to rescue me from the abusive family life I lived. They made me feel so special and welcomed me by making my favorite meals or taking me to their favorite restaurants. I would go to church with Jan and her family, where I knew they were praying hard for me. None of these families were perfect, but above all else, there was love and comfort—two things I didn't have much of in my home.

I used the positivity around me and even the negativity as fuel to become the best version of me that I could. I started getting involved in different sports and activities in school, and I was succeeding. As expected, my stepfather continued to ignore my accomplishments, but I almost made it a game. The better I did, the more he looked like an ass to everyone around him by doing the opposite of what a parent should do when a child has success. In today's world, we call that, "give them a reason to hate." Still, I was suffering—mentally, emotionally, and physically.

Chapter 4

MOM

I was far from the only one breaking under the physical, mental, and emotional strain. My mom was going through some medical issues as they discovered endometriosis, likely exacerbated by the amount of stress she was exposed to by her husband and stepchildren.

I recall my stepfather's behavior was the cause of ninety-nine percent of the arguments between the two of them. He acted like his boys were entitled to whatever they wanted, while us ladies were entitled to nothing. We were treated like we were the lucky ones to be in HIS house. And he always reminded us we were just guests and nothing more. How is that a marriage? How must my mother have felt, knowing she brought us into the house. To her, there was no turning back. She had a husband and three daughters. This was her life. Where would she go? What would she do?

My mother stood her ground best she could. She did what she had to do to make sure everything remained as even as possible between the boys and the girls. There was a day where I wanted to help the boys cut the lawn. I ran outside excitedly, but my mother was not going to have any of that. She yelled for me to get in the house immediately when she saw me pushing the mower. She told me that was their job, and I was not helping them do it. She told me I could help with the lawn when they helped me do the dishes or clean the house.

Another time, when it snowed, I barely had my second boot on when she told me I was not going outside to shovel. That was *not* my job, and she continued to remind me of it. We were very unionized in my home. I understand her point now, but at the time I was thinking it would be nice if we could all be on the same team for once. We couldn't. It was impossible. But I still had the optimism of a child, with the ability to see circumstances in an entirely different light than what they actually were. Adults often lose that ability. My mom had lost it. This was her, and consequently my, reality.

Still, my mom tried to make the best out of tense or bad situations. She tried to make Sunday dinners a time for the family to come together. She tried to make holidays joyful. She made efforts to spend quality time with me outside of the reach of my stepfather's imposing glare or loud silence. She took me on shopping trips and road trips through the city to escape the anxieties that permeated our home. She supported me in so many ways, both large and small, but she was hopelessly overpowered when it came to the those awaiting us at the dinner table, desperate to break me down.

I think the natural tendency is to show outrage and fury toward my mother for not protecting me and for allowing me to be abused physically and emotionally, but not all of it can be laid at her feet. She made every effort to pull a blended family together that had unique and, at times, very toxic traits of their own construction. She didn't submit to her husband. In fact, she fought, she yelled, she kicked and screamed, but it didn't matter. There were consequences to not submitting. He had total control over her, despite any resistance from her. This is the mind of an abuse victim. It is based in fear—fear of repercussions, fear for children, fear for your very life. It alters how you make decisions and your actions.

I know she has guilt about what went on, but I am not sure she even remembers the extent of it. I think to myself that if I was traumatized enough to block out so much of it, what has her mind done over the years to protect her? Some of it will come as a surprise to her as she reads this book, due to her state of mind. She was an adult, but also a victim of abuse. Because I recognized that, even from an early age, I didn't dare go crying to her about what went on while she wasn't around to see it. I knew it would only put her in a position to have to defend me, and the intense and scary cycle of abuse would start all over. There would always be consequences. She knew it, and I was quickly learning.

Mom would "run away from home" periodically just to escape the stress. As I grew into an adult, I started to understand how and why. She just hated him so much, but she couldn't say that out loud. At times, she simply couldn't handle staying there—the stress was killing her.

A few of the times she "ran away," I remember feeling scared and alone. She probably felt that I was at least physically safe with my stepfather for just one night, and I was, but I didn't know that at the time. He hated me, as far as I knew. And even sensing my fear wouldn't bring out any humanity in this man. He would continue to ignore me, leaving me in my own thoughts and utter silence. I would spend the entire time in my bedroom just to be invisible until my dad would pick me up the very next day—noon, every Saturday, like clockwork—the best day of each week.

Chapter 5

DAD

Once there was a little red ant. Trying to move a rubber tree plant. But everyone knows an ant, can't, move a rubber tree plant. But he has high hopes …

Every Sunday, when my dad and his girlfriend (soon-to-be bride) would drive me back home after a fun filled, quality time together weekend, we would sing in the car from Chicago to the suburbs. We'd all giggle as we extended some of the words to see how long we could make them (*movvvvve, hiiiiighhhh*).

In my opinion, my dad walked on water. When I was with him, I was loved; I was cared for. I didn't have to be anything other than the little girl I was. And I was definitely not ignored or looked upon with disgust. I looked forward to our time together more than almost anything. Looking back, it amazes me that I didn't want a lot of toys or television or big, extravagant trips. What I was desperately longing for was simply to have the freedom to be a little girl and be loved for it. Not so much of an ask.

When we were together, we would often spend time at my grandmother's house, so he could cut her lawn or take care of her "to do" list. I loved spending time with her and with my aunts, uncles, and cousins. My dad would help me with my homework, we would play catch or cards, watch TV, and do household chores together. We were joined at the hip for the 36 hours he had me every week. He was so relaxed and happy. My weekends were filled with love, interest, and support. It was exactly what I needed to balance out the abuse I endured all week long.

As an extra bonus, we would also visit my sister, her new husband, and her beautiful baby on the way to my dad's house in the city. My sister and her husband lived with his mom and dad in another suburb. This was another highlight of my weekend. I loved my sister and missed her (and her unending protection) terribly. But time was made up quickly when I saw her, and my new niece became the love of my life. I was only ten years old when she was born, so it was like I had my own live doll to play with.

I spent every Saturday and half of Sunday with my dad until I was sixteen years old. At sixteen, our visits shifted to every other weekend. And then, at eighteen, I had my own apartment. But through it all, he called me every day of the week to see how my day was, tell me he loved me, tell me how wonderful I was, and tell me how I made him so proud. He was always respectful. He opened my car doors, the house doors, and would tell me, "This is how you should always be treated. This is how a gentleman will treat you one day." Decades later, I won't settle for anything less.

My dad married his new wife when I was fourteen years old, but they had been together since I was six. Throughout that time, and even the first several years they were married, she treated me as if I were her own blood. She lived in Wrigleyville, a very trendy area of the city before they married, and we had spent a lot of our weekend time there. We would have our own time together, reading books, singing songs, and getting dressed up together for my dad to take us out on our date nights.

As I grew older, my stepmom became a beacon of light in my life. Knowing I struggled with comprehension, she would spend hours with me every weekend reading. We read the entire book *The Lion, the Witch and the Wardrobe* at one point. Her patience with me during that time was unfaltering. She would also help me with my homework every week, rub and tickle my back, and sing whatever songs I wanted in the car. She was kind and good spirited. And she made my dad happy. What else could I ask for?

Everything was so great and easy with them … except I had a secret. I never told them about the abuse I was enduring at home. So, they couldn't intervene or take me to live with them. They had no idea there was even an issue at all. Even as a young girl, I was more worried about others than myself. I didn't want them to worry about me. I didn't want them to be mad at my mom. I didn't want fights or ugly battles. Most of all, I did not want to be the cause of what could possibly happen if my dad knew any of this. My time with my dad was a time when I felt simple love and security—I wanted to soak in every second, not taint it with something ugly. And honestly, I really did think my mom was doing the best she could, and that she had very little idea, until this book, what was going on at home while she worked full-time.

It wasn't until my mid-teens that I told my dad and stepmom that I was being mistreated by my stepfather and the boys. And by that time, I started putting up my front. I downplayed it. I pretended I wasn't bothered by the abuse at all. In fact, I would never even say the word "abuse." I just acknowledged it and brushed it off, like it was an inconvenience. It was so much more, of course, but again, I was a teenager coping the best way I could.

When I did finally tell my dad and stepmom what things were like, they weren't completely shocked. They told me that on all those car rides driving home on Sunday evenings, singing all those songs, I would always clam up about five minutes from home. They said my personality changed instantly each time. They thought I was being my usual thoughtful self and didn't want my mom to see us having so much fun together. But I was subconsciously going back to the place I needed to be to survive the next five days.

They felt awful that, for all those years, they had no idea what was really going on. And each Sunday night, we would pull into our driveway, I would get out of their car, hug and kiss them goodbye, walk inside and pass my mom in the family room, say, "Goodnight," as I kept walking to my bedroom, close the door, and wave out the window, as tears rolled endlessly down my wet cheeks. They wouldn't drive away until they saw me waving. Of course, from that distance, they couldn't see that I was crying as I was waving to them. As a mom today, that memory makes me so sad. I felt utterly alone. I was also completely unaware that the dynamics of that relationship would also soon change. What was once my haven—the place I could escape my reality—became something else entirely.

The once tight relationship I had with my stepmom turned into something else over time. Slowly at first, as she started picking up a bottle of alcohol which seemed to be more frequently and at odd times, and then more so, as her drinking increased. Watching this beautiful, compassionate, intelligent woman deteriorate was incredibly sad. She had started drinking at some point after they married and she moved into the house with my middle sister, who was already there and had long since marked her territory. I watched how little time it took for my sister to destroy my stepmom's good spirit and positive outlook, just like she had mine.

While "normal" teenagers (oxymoron at its finest there) rebel against their parents and authority, my sister took it to the extreme. It seemed like she thrived in spreading chaos, destruction, and drama wherever she went. And I, unfortunately, had to watch it for much of my life. I spent even more time at my dad's house on spring and summer breaks, so I saw firsthand how she treated them. She refused to go to college or get a job, so she would sit home, eat, leave her dirty dishes on the counter, and watch TV—all day long.

When my dad and stepmom would arrive home from work, she would yell at them for making noise and because she couldn't hear the TV. She would yell at them for opening the blinds that she had drawn all day. If they asked about the dishes, she'd tell them she'd do it when she felt like it. She would blatantly dare my dad to take my stepmom's side. She seemed to have no regard or respect for my dad, and definitely none for my stepmom. Even on Father's Day, she would leave the house and spend the day with a friend or a boyfriend's family. It was some of the most despicable, disrespectful behavior I have ever seen, even as an adult.

These malicious tendencies eventually played a part in destroying my father's happy relationship– slowly turning his beautiful wife, my adoring stepmom into someone I no longer recognized. And then, there was more stress, as my elderly grandmother moved into their home to live full-time. My dad was so preoccupied with my grandmother and trying to keep my sister in school, and off drugs, he could no longer maintain a healthy marriage. He did the best he could. He loved all of us so much. But in the end, it just wasn't enough. His health suffered from all the stress and before we knew it, he was in the hospital for a triple bypass.

When we found out that my dad's chances of surviving the surgery were less than favorable, I thought I would lose my mind. Not to sound so cliché, but he was my rock. He was my world. He was the only man in my life who loved me, wanted the best for me, showed respect toward me, and most of all, protected me. I couldn't bare the thought of losing him. But dad had other plans. As a first-generation Italian, born and raised in Chicago, semi-pro boxer in college, and Army veteran, my dad proved far tougher than his bleak medical prognosis would indicate. He did survive. And he took it as the warning it was.

He stopped smoking and started eating healthier than ever. He incorporated a workout routine and stuck to it day in and day out. He understood then how stress could kill him, so he did his best not to let so many things bother him. The stress continued, of course, despite his best intentions. The situations with his mother, wife, and daughter all continued to play out in a downward spiral in which he was the center.

As for me, I took that warning as a wake-up call for myself. I started to appreciate him even more (if that was possible), trying to spend as much time with him and support him as much as I could. My stepmom also made some changes. She knew that staying away from stress sadly meant staying away from my sister. So, she took matters into her own hands. She hired a moving company to pack up all my sister's things and move them into a storage unit that was paid for thirty days. And then, she changed the locks on the house! This all happened quickly one morning while my sister was out. It was brilliant. At that point, my sister was twenty-four years old. Enough was enough.

Chapter 6

NEW BEGINNINGS

"I'm outta here! As soon as I can do it, I am moving out," said my sixteen-year-old self. Yes, while other teenagers are planning what they're wearing to prom or studying for an exam, I was constructing an escape plan. I was in my high school counselor's office by the end of sophomore year to find out how many credits I had and what I needed to do to graduate early. I started to realize that, despite how powerless I felt in my home, I did have some control over my life. I could decide how the next couple of years played out … if I started preparing. So, a plan was exactly what I made.

I worked insanely hard and was able to graduate high school six months early. My friends thought I was crazy missing out on the last half of senior year, but I didn't feel like I would miss out on anything but extra homework, so it was fine with me. But more importantly, the sooner I could get done, the sooner I could move on with my life. The sooner I could take the control I was desperately needing to take.

I also had been working various jobs since I was fifteen, saving money for my plan to get out. I worked at a movie theater, a drive-in theater, and different stores in our local mall. Some of those jobs were seasonal, others I worked simultaneously. I had enough money to buy my first car, a Chevy Chevette, which I affectionately referred to as, "My Vette." After all, I would need to be able to drive to my new full-time job as a travel agent, while I waited for classes to start at Harper Community College.

I approached my mom a few months before my eighteenth birthday about moving out on my own. She didn't even try to talk me out of it, even though I was only seventeen. Not only did she not try to talk me out of it, but she also went with me to look at several places. I think, on some level, she knew I needed to get out of that house almost as much as I did. Soon, I found the perfect place! I signed the lease and moved in as soon as I turned eighteen. I had already established credit, so I didn't even need a co-signer. Besides, my parent's made it clear they were not co-signing for me. Not for a car, not for an apartment, not for anything. I was on my own. I was eighteen.

I was making just enough money at that time to budget for food, my car payment, rent, and a credit card bill for furniture I bought. I was offered hand-me-down furniture from other family members, but I wanted my place to look nice and new. I needed my own fresh start, and I wanted it to be on my terms.

After nine years of living, surviving, and at times, thriving in one of the most toxic, dysfunctional environments imaginable, I finally escaped. But a physical escape is often easier than a mental and emotional one. The long-term effects lingered and shaped me for far longer than I could have possibly understood at the time. What transpired after I moved out of that house, at a time when I finally thought I was taking some control back, part of me will never understand. Although, when I remember I was only a teenager at the time, impacted by years of abuse, I guess it's not that difficult to understand after all.

I have heard unhealed childhood trauma causes numerous adult issues—everything from people pleasing to feelings of abandonment. Anyone who has watched a Lifetime Channel movie or has even the most basic understanding of psychology, understands that no matter how much abuse someone endures from a family member, particularly a parent, that person will crave love and affection from the very people who tormented them. I wish I could claim to be the exception to this rule, but I simply cannot.

Despite years of accumulated mental abuse, bullying, and even physical violence, somehow, I managed to strive not only for the approval of my abusive stepfather of mine, but also my stepbrothers. I could not wrap my brain around it. I knew, without a doubt, their behavior was wrong. I knew I hated them all. I had my guard up for years. Yet I still somehow found myself seeking their approval—all of them, for so many years.

I would actually have conversations with myself, recognizing that my behavior made no logical sense, but I was unable to change it. I would ask myself why I was acting this way. Why would I care, one way or another, what they thought about me? In my mind, they were all abusive. In my mind, they were all sick fucks—each one of them in their own way.

For years, this conversation went on in my head. And at end of each one, regardless of what I told myself, I still wanted to please them. I still wanted them to like me. I still wanted them to accept me as a daughter and sister. As I look back, I cannot explain why I was seeking their approval or acceptance, but I could not stop.

Despite my plan, the relief of getting out of the house of horrors, and the excitement of my new independence, being on my own was much harder than I thought it would be. I was just starting at Harper Community College full-time, and I had started working three jobs in order to pay all of my new expenses, which started to add up quickly. I was now cleaning houses, working at a gym, and an assistant to an entrepreneur I had met while cleaning her house. She really liked me and offered me the position. She also took me under her wing and became one of my first true mentors. She taught me a lot about being an entrepreneur and business, and I will always be grateful for that.

This was also right around the time my father had his triple bypass, bringing with it an avalanche of emotions for me. My dad had always put a huge emphasis on college. I was going to be his only child to attend, so he had high hopes for me. And I never wanted to let him down, especially while he was fighting for his new chance at life.

He knew how ambitious I was. Eventually, he saw what I had to overcome throughout my childhood, and he knew I could do it. Even during my years at Harper Community College, he helped me with my homework. He was a master at math, accounting, and business. This was another way we bonded. He was so proud of me!

I would still go to his house on the weekends, have dinner with him, and meet him for breakfast on Sunday mornings. We were still as close as we were when he had me on the weekends as a child. We were washing our cars together and sharing stories of his younger years. But soon, I didn't have as much time as I once did. And the decisions I would make over the next few years broke my dad's heart.

Chapter 7

FIRST LOVE

During my time at Harper, I was busy, to say the least. I was going to school full-time, studying, doing well in my classes, and working three jobs to pay for my rent, car, and other bills. I was busy, but okay. In fact, I have always tended to thrive under pressure. I scheduled time for everything … everything except fun. But that all changed in my last year at Harper, when I fell in love with a boy. His name was Joey. He was not a college student, but a blue-collar worker—a baggage handler at a major airline, with no college degree. He was a co-worker and friend of one of my stepbrothers, who introduced us, and within a few short months, he moved in with me. While blinded by young love, I was also very practical—I needed help paying my rent.

My father, on the other hand, was not happy. As far as he was concerned, Joey already had three strikes against him. First, he was a blue-collar worker. Second, he did not have a college degree. And third, he lived with me out of wedlock. My dad made his disapproval very clear, and it worked, to an extent. I felt horribly guilty. You see, no one does guilt quite like Catholics, and Italian Catholics have elevated it to an artform.

Living with a man before marriage was unacceptable to my father. He told me he was embarrassed about what our family and friends would think. With the Italians, image is everything. I was his only daughter that actually had a fighting chance to set herself up for success and he thought this would interfere with that path. My dad never said he thought I was a whore but seeing how disappointed in me he was made me feel like it. I was so young. And with this young mentality, I thought I had to fix it. I didn't want my dad to be embarrassed. I needed to justify my decision of living with a man *and* prove that I was not a whore. The answer? Marriage.

After Joey proposed to me, I immediately questioned whether he asked my dad for approval. It hadn't even occurred to him. He was only twenty years old and was never taught these types of things. *Well,* I thought, *there's another strike.* But, to his credit, he went to my dad's house to ask for permission to marry me. My dad had heard about this upcoming visit, so I think he had his speech already prepared. As soon as Joey arrived, my dad asked my stepmom to pour them a scotch and asked us ladies to leave the room. Then Joey got the lecture you'd expect. I heard it started with, "If you ever mistreat my daughter…"

As soon as we got in the car to go home, Joey wiped sweat off his forehead and said, straight faced, "That was bullshit!" But, to me, it needed to be done. And the wedding plans began!

My mother, on the other hand, was a different story. She backed my decision. She always did. She knew that I was strong enough to recover from any bad decision I ever made. She was ecstatic, as she knew how much I loved this young man. She loved him too. During this period in time, you couldn't *not* love him, he was amazing. At this early stage of his life, he did not have one enemy because he had the unique ability to captivate everyone's attention with his charisma and positive energy. Everyone wanted to be his friend. He made me very happy, and my mom saw that for the first time in years.

Not only did Joey make me and my mom happy, but our relationship made my stepfather and stepbrothers happy, too. Why I cared even slightly about their happiness is something I still can barely wrap my head around. My childhood home life involved mental, emotional, and physical abuse by these people, and still, I felt a need to get their approval. Somehow, my new fiancé fit the bill. Looking back, I am not sure how I could have ever thought that someone who my stepdad and my stepbrothers loved was the ideal man for me, but again … I was nineteen, with nineteen-year-old thoughts and emotions.

Joey did love me, and we had a ton of fun together. Our relationship gave me some light and ease that I hadn't had before. It gave me some fun and laughter back in an otherwise busy, work-filled life. Joey was showing me positive energy, care, love, and compassion, which I had only ever seen by my father and only on weekends growing up. But despite his love for me, in retrospect, I don't think Joey would have actually proposed if it wasn't for me needing my dad's approval.

This approval wasn't as easy to get as I had thought though. The disappointment was overwhelming for my dad. He had something completely different in mind for my future—something completely different than having his nineteen-year-old daughter get married. He wanted to see me graduate from college, get an important job, and climb the corporate ladder. He wanted to see me as the independent woman he knew I was (way before I truly knew it). He thought playing the "wifey" role was way below my caliber, especially since according to him, I was "too young" to be a wife in the first place.

He didn't know I was only trying to prove to him that I wasn't a whore (my word, not his). He didn't understand that I had been swimming in a sea of craving approval and acceptance from unworthy, toxic men for most of my life. How could he possibly understand? It's hard for me to understand. But what he thought he did understand was that my future would be ruined if I took this path. He begged me not to do it, but the irony is that my relentless desire for his approval outweighed his happiness.

When he couldn't convince me to change my mind, my dad decided to pull the "money and financial support card," telling me that if I took this path, he would no longer pay for my college tuition. And he most certainly would not pay for my wedding. Yet how many of these threatening tactics actually work with teenagers? Not many, if you know teenagers. I fell into this category and dug my heels in deeper. I have rarely been accused of not being resourceful. And within two weeks, I solved the college tuition problem. I found a full-time office job that offered 100% college reimbursement. My wedding plans continued!

My dad could not believe I was going to go through with this wedding, despite all his attempts to the contrary. He told me that it would take me forever to finish college at a part-time pace. He was afraid I would like the money from a job too much and not have incentive to finish my education. This made me more bound and determined to take the challenge and beat the odds. I had to prove to him and everyone else who doubted me that I was strong and had the ability to make my own decisions. But to him, I was making one bad decision after another.

I landed an entry level position at a cell phone company, Cellular One, in Schaumburg, Illinois, which opened the door to a sales position at a candy company, Leaf, Inc., in Lake Forest, Illinois. Entry level or not, I learned a ton from these positions, even information that helped me make it through my college business classes. That's the key through life though, always take something valuable out of every experience. That's what I did at these beginning jobs.

And all the while, my wedding planning season was moving full force ahead. My mom and I were having so much fun. We loved looking forward to something so positive. During this time, I drew much closer to her. We shopped for gorgeous wedding gowns together, picked the venue together, decided on the menu together, and tasted delicious pastries for the sweets table together. We found something fun to talk about or do every single day.

Even the situation between my mom and stepfather was getting better. I believe that since he and my stepbrothers were treating me better than ever before, it took a lot of pressure off her always having to fix things between us or unjustifiably have to defend me for some ridiculous claim or another. As crazy as it may seem, I even became close to most of my stepbrothers. At this point, we all became friends. They were all friends with Joey already, so we started hanging out together. The past was never discussed and living in the peace I had been searching for my whole life, I was able to put the mental torture that they all inflicted for so many years behind me.

Yay me! I thought this was great. I learned how to forgive! They loved me now because they loved my fiancé! I didn't care *why* they were treating me great. I was just happy they were. As time went on, I realized I had not forgiven them at all. I was just suppressing my feelings because things finally seemed to be better … at least on that front.

Unfortunately, as those relationships were quickly improving, my relationships with my dad and stepmom were deteriorating just as fast. They made no secret their disapproval of this wedding, and no matter what I said or did, they could not get onboard. Still, because they were who they were, they helped sometimes in the planning, and even paid for some things. But deep down, they were completely heartbroken I was taking this path. I was not quite sure of how their marriage was at the time or if my stepmom was still drinking so heavily. I felt deliriously happy for the first true time in my life, and I wasn't going to let anyone or anything change that.

I was only thinking of myself. I felt like I finally won the approval of all the men in my life who I thought mistreated me, abused me mentally, physically, verbally and spiritually! God Bless. Quite an accomplishment on my end, I thought. I was also *eating up* the approval and acceptance I had been seeking my whole life by the people I should have cared the least about. So, I allowed my dad and stepmom to take a backseat to all the fun. I didn't see it at the time, but I did later. They had every reason to be hurt. I was mesmerized by the approval and acceptance of the people who hurt me most, while simultaneously hurting the ones who loved me most. The term "childhood trauma" wasn't even a term yet.

Chapter 8

HERE COMES THE BRIDE

About six months before our wedding day, I was diagnosed with a tumor in my brain's pituitary gland. Naturally, this was a huge blow to me and to my parents. No one really understood what to expect—this was a rare condition, and I was very young. A few months passed before we could get a prognosis and develop a strategy to maintain the tumor, while trying to avoid removing it through a high-risk surgery. However, the tumor itself created risks. I was in danger of losing my eyesight and I had stopped ovulating. I worked with an endocrinologist who, by trial and error, played around with a dosage of the meds that would shrink the tumor to a manageable size, so that I would not lose my eyesight, and so I could possibly start to ovulate again.

The doctors mentioned the "no baby scenario" early on during the strategy phase, but I was so young, I wasn't really concerned about it. After everything I had been through as a child, I never imagined God would ever bless me with a child of my own anyway. And even though I was now on good terms with my stepfather and stepbrothers, I would never forget the promises I had already made to myself hundreds of times that I would never allow them to see my kids if I had any. So, part of me thought it might just be easier.

Easier for me didn't mean easier all around though. I recognized that Joey wanted children very badly, and I felt badly about not being able to give him that. I felt like it was the right thing to do to give him an out. After all, no ovulation means no babies. I'll never forget our conversation because as much as he said he wanted to be a father one day, he said he wanted me more. He didn't care if I couldn't get pregnant and even mentioned that we could always adopt one day. His only concern was for my health. His response truly touched me. He would rather stick with me, even if it meant giving up a dream of his own. I had never felt so loved and secure.

So, at a time when the most important relationship of my life—my relationship with my dad—had taken a dive, I was also diagnosed with a brain tumor, told I'd probably never have children, and was planning a wedding. I was stressed, to say the least. I was also working full time. And let's not forget, I was also not even twenty years old yet. This was also a time when I allowed people close to me get in my head and tell me I was too young to get married. Some friends and family told me I was making a big mistake, and that weighed heavily on me. As an avoidance mechanism, even with everything else going on, I thought it would be the perfect time to enroll in my undergraduate program! I had just graduated from Harper with my associates degree and wanted to pursue my bachelor's degree. I had the option to take the first semester off because of the wedding, but that's just not my style.

As I continued to work my way through my medical treatments and plan the wedding, my dad, stepmom, and I began building our relationship back up. To my extreme delight, they started to get involved in the wedding plans. As soon as they jumped onboard, I got them caught up on all the details. Either they were truly having fun with it, or they put on a good show because it felt like things were right back to normal with us. And I was never so relieved in my life. I think they knew they were either going to be with me, or against me because this wedding was happening. So, much to my relief, they were going to be with me.

They became very involved with the church details. My stepmom was going to sing at the church, so we spent time a lot of time together picking out the perfect music for her, as well as psalms for the speakers. And my dad had only two demands for after the church … top-shelf liquor at the reception and great music for dancing!

As the wedding planning marched forward, I was becoming more excited and was getting closer to friends and family who were standing up. I was feeling so good that I even asked my middle sister to stand up in my wedding. Initially, she accepted, but then she became pregnant and changed her mind. To some that knew our family dynamics best, they thought she did it on purpose during my wedding planning because she hated any attention on me. But I never even thought that because I honestly didn't give a shit what she did or didn't do or why. I was having the time of my life—her pregnancy was not going to interfere in any way. I was happy for her though, hoping the baby would soften her and somehow transform her into a pleasant person. Unfortunately, I was wrong. She was due about two months after my wedding, so she insisted that the best time to have a baby shower was the week before my wedding. And the baby shower went as she wished.

I spent the night before my wedding at my dad and stepmom's house. They went above and beyond to make me feel special. They completely pampered me with new décor in the spare bedroom—beautiful white eye-lit bedding and lace tulle. They had soaps and lotions and scented candles for relaxation. We stayed up that night reminiscing about the great weekends we spent together my entire life … we may have even sung those old songs again.

Then they gave me the gift I never thought I'd get. They told me how proud they were of me and how much faith they had in me. They told me they knew I would be a great wife and that I would do whatever I set my mind to because I was the strongest and most determined person they knew. I felt like the luckiest girl in the world. I had the best dad and stepmom a girl could ever have.

Morning came and I went to my mom's house to get ready. It was pouring down rain, but that didn't stop the excitement we all felt. It was one of the happiest days I had ever experienced in that house. My friends, family, and bridesmaids were there sharing in my joy, and the photographer was snapping away, capturing what should be treasured memories for a lifetime. The fact that I was happy there was one thing, but the fact that I had friends there completely another. Due to the unhealthy circumstances of my upbringing, it wasn't typical for me to have friends over as I grew up. But I tried hard not to focus on that on my special day.

My dad came to the door just before I was finished getting ready because he realized I forgot something at his house. It was at this moment that both my mother and I realized that we never invited him to the house for the pre-wedding snacks and photos. This definitely impacted my mood, but it was such a crazy busy day and the cameras started snapping and lights started flashing that I did not have time to dwell on it or fix it.

To make matters worse, the photographer had no idea that my true dad wasn't there and kept calling for Bride and Father of the Bride photos. I was sick to my stomach posing with my stepfather. Yes, I had forgiven him on the surface for the way he treated me growing up, but he absolutely had not earned the right to have any photo taken with me on my special day! My forgiveness was only on the surface. On the inside, I still despised him and everything he had done.

To this day, I still think about how badly I felt that my own dad was not there that morning and afternoon. He should have been there while I was getting ready. He should have been there while the fun and pre-celebrations were going on. He should have been the VERY first person to take a picture with me that day. We barely discussed this. My parents did not have a great relationship, so I am not sure they would have felt comfortable anyway. I don't think I will ever forgive myself for missing this detail.

Before we knew it, the flashes stopped, and three shiny black limos pulled up to the house to transport all twelve bridesmaids, mothers, and grandmothers to the church. The song, "Going to the Chapel," was playing and everyone was singing along, making me feel so special. But all I could think about was my dad, and how his feelings were probably already hurt. I knew it was only going to get worse when those wedding photo proofs showed up in a few weeks. But this was my wedding day, and I knew I had one shot at making today the best day of my life. So, I tried to put those negative feelings out of my head while on the way to the church. I played along with all the festivities and started getting really excited! We had a blast in the limo, and when we arrived at the church, my bridesmaids whisked me away into the private bride's room.

Within minutes, the door opened, and in walked my handsome dad. Every single woman in the room with me, there were over a dozen, started bawling. For the first time in my life, I saw my dad cry—uncontrollably. It was the most emotional moment I had ever experienced in my life. He was so sweet and sincere. All I can remember him saying over and over is, "My baby!"

After everyone was seated, my dad and I made our way to the church doors. My dad looked at me, put his hands on my face and told me, "It is not too late. You do not have to do this." I was shocked. This was the kind of thing you only see in the movies! He continued, "I do not care how many people are in there right now. We can turn around right now, and you can say you had a change of heart. You wouldn't disappoint anyone. Everyone will understand."

I stared at him in disbelief, but I knew it was coming from a place of love and protection.

"Here Comes the Bride" started playing on the organ. The church doors opened. We took one final look at each other, smiled, and took a step forward.

Chapter 9

AFTER THE LOVIN

The Father/Daughter dance was beautiful and heartfelt. I surprised my dad with the song by Engelbert Humperdinck, "After the Lovin." He used to sing it to me when I was a little girl, rocking me slowly in his arms. I never forgot those times … or that song (and never, ever will). I mean how could I? It was those special times with my dad that I held onto with everything I had while I was growing up.

His expression when the DJ started a few chords of "Daddy's Little Girl," then mixed right into "After the Lovin" was priceless. I will never forget that look and how tight he held me during that dance. We swirled around on the dance floor together, me safe and protected in his loving arms, just like I always felt whenever I was close to him. I truly was Daddy's Little Girl and always would be. He looked at me just like he did my whole life, like I was his little princess and there is nothing in the world he wouldn't do for me. A tear slid down his cheek. And of course, I was sobbing like a baby. He said all the right things to me within those few minutes. All the right things that I will remember for the rest of my life.

In one of those cruel life ironies, the videographer ran out of tape just as "After the Lovin," started, missing the whole thing. I didn't know it then but could not believe it when I found out later. I was pissed. But the cruelest irony of the night was to come on the same dance floor, after the videographer had finally reloaded his camera. Later that night, Bette Midler's "The Wind Beneath My Wings" started playing.

I'm not sure who encouraged me to dance with my stepfather for this song, and I drank too much champagne to remember exactly how it happened, but the videographer, once again didn't miss a beat with mine and his interactions. The fucking idiot was catching every second of this surreal moment—but not in the surreal way you would expect at a wedding—surreal as in I could not believe this was happening *on my special day*. And seriously, "Wind Beneath My Wings"—there couldn't be a song that did not represent our relationship any more than that one. I never, ever felt like he supported me. All he did was weigh me down, not help me fly.

To make matters worse, my stepfather decided to take this opportunity to apologize for the way he treated me all those years, right then and there, on my wedding dancefloor. He was sincere, he was detailed, and he was sorry. Needless to say, I broke down, along with everyone else in the room who knew the rocky relationship we had always had. I was so completely and utterly torn up emotionally. This was something I never expected to happen. Not ever. But at the same time, I also felt cheated. This was my day, my time, and he was robbing me of that too. This was not the time and certainly not the place to do this. Then again, he was never the brightest person in the room.

I knew I deserved better than that. Some of the friends and family who were there and saw it all were so happy. They pulled me aside, hugging me, and wiping tears of joy from their faces, telling me, "Isn't it great that he acknowledged his horrific behavior and apologized for it?"

And the answer would be, "Yeah, I guess, sure. But then and there on my wedding day?"

This moment should have had its own scene, nowhere near what was supposed to be one of the happiest days of my life. He should not have been given the opportunity to bury his apology while I was distracted by my own wedding, not to mention, a little drunk besides. I deserved better than that. And I wanted to focus on the men in my life who added value, not take it away, such as my new husband and my dad. This was not a time for him. Plain and simple. And unfortunately, I could never truly understand if he did it authentically or if he did it to rob me of one more happiness.

My feelings did not have a chance to be validated as he wedged his apology in between the garter toss and the chicken dance. I should have, at a minimum, had a chance to prepare for this assault on my emotions on an already emotionally charged day. As a result, I said nothing to him. Nothing in return to him that day on the dance floor, except for, "thank you." I couldn't even gather enough coherent thoughts to consider what I would have wanted to say to him in that instance. Protect my mom's feelings and accept his apology or tell him to fuck off because it was a little too little and a lot too late.

And just like that…we moved on. *After all, what else could we do?*

Chapter 10

SURPRISE!

The next couple of years of my life were absolutely everything that a young woman hopelessly in love could wish for. At the young age of twenty-one, I was working full time for a company that offered 100% college reimbursement, while taking two or three night classes at a time. My husband and I excitedly purchased our first home. It was a townhome and the perfect place for us to establish our roots. We also knew we'd eventually want something more, so we started saving money for a bigger home.

During this time, we were traveling constantly, as he still worked for a major airline at the time. We were fortunate enough to travel on thirteen different long weekend trips within the first year of our marriage. We would often travel with his softball team, and after the games, we'd have a few beers and socialize with our softball family. Joey always put me on a pedestal, bragging to everyone how I was the best cook and how well I took care of him. He made me feel so special—so secure and valued. He genuinely seemed grateful and proud to be with me.

It struck me how different an experience this was compared to how I had been treated by most men in my life. He made me want to be the best wife I could be and take care of him as best I could—not because I had to, but because I wanted to. He helped to bring my confidence to the next level. He made me want to match his positive energy, and soon, I did. I was the happiest I could ever remember being. My marriage was like nothing I had ever seen close up. We were friends, and we always had fun together. I seriously felt like I married my best friend (because I did). Sometimes, the two of us would head to the airport with only bathing suits in our luggage and see what flights we could jump on stand-by. We were living our best lives!

As time went on, my studies became increasingly challenging, and money became tighter. We had to make changes and start being more responsible—we had to start "adulting." So, the workload increased (along with the stress), and the traveling eventually slowed … at least for me.

On top of taking two to three college courses and working full-time, I was also taking on all the household chores and responsibilities in the townhouse. While Joey worked hard, he also fully supported the saying, *work hard, play hard.* He was then on three softball leagues, golfed on every one of his days off, and started going out after work every night for drinks. I felt like one of us was growing up, but the other one wasn't.

As hard as we worked, we weren't saving any money at all. In fact, it was just the opposite because of all the expenses of going out all the time. While I watched the balance in our bank account dwindle to near nothing, I tried explaining to him that we needed to make some changes. I tried to explain to him that he couldn't go out every night after work. I started to feel more like we had a mother-son relationship than a husband-wife relationship. And as a child would do, he became extremely defiant, doing anything and everything he could to irritate me even further. I never did find out what triggered this, but I was getting fed up. We started spending less and less time together and inevitably, started growing apart.

After about a year of us going in completely different directions, I confided in my friend Marlene. She was shocked but didn't have a lot of advice on the matter. How could I make my husband do what he was supposed to do as a homeowner and a husband? I couldn't. He was acting like a teenager. And sadly, I became his mother. Marlene was supportive, especially when I told her I was considering divorcing Joey, knowing full well that I could not live like this for the rest of my life. This was not what I expected out of him or our relationship. I deserved more. We used to have so much fun together when we were partying and blowing money and traveling all over the country. I began to question if it wasn't really *me* he had been enjoying, but all the fun instead.

So, here I was having marital problems, working my full-time job, and going to school. I may have been a little less than friendly to co-workers (to say the least). I couldn't help it—my patience level was short, and my attitude was, looking back, embarrassing. One day, I was having a conversation with our C-Level manager who had recently come to town to check on how our department was doing. Out of the blue, he said, "You are pregnant."

I laughed and said, "That's actually impossible."

He said, "I have four children. I know when a woman is pregnant. You have been a different person this visit, and I can see it in your face."

Now, even back then, this type of conversation could have cost him his job, so I was a little thrown off. But because I knew him, and his outspoken, push the envelope, sparkling personality, I wasn't offended. I just thought it was him being himself.

Our entire department went to lunch that day, and on our way back to our cars, I had one of the most surreal experiences of my life. All five of us followed this manager into Walgreens, where he shockingly walked me to the feminine care product aisle. Once there, he asked me to pick out a pregnancy test.

"It's on me. You need to know for your own safety."

It was one thing to make a comment and ask me about being pregnant. This was completely overstepping his bounds and a total violation of privacy. I was shocked. Still, I tried to explain to him, although it was none of his business, the reason I knew I could not be pregnant. And, of course, I now had an audience—my entire department. To this day, I still cannot believe this really happened. They all listened to my explanation, but I do not recall any one of them trying to intervene or get him to back off. He could make or break anyone of us and our careers, so we just did what he said. I humored him. Off we went with a double pack of whatever brand it was.

The box sat on my desk for the next several hours, while everyone in my department stopped by periodically to see if I took the test, perpetuating this unbelievable lack of privacy. I didn't have to pee, or maybe I didn't want to know. I did feel like I had the flu the day before, and I was tired. I also was craving turkey, stuffing, and mashed potatoes, fiercely, and it was the month of August, so I thought that was weird. I also had not had a period in a while, but I wasn't keeping track. And nothing had changed from my last doctor's appointment, so I was in denial. I am not sure, but at about 3:30 p.m. that day, the "signs" started to outweigh my logic. I stepped away from my desk, box in hand, and went into the bathroom.

Immediately, the tell-tale sign of pregnancy—two pink, parallel lines—showed up. Still in disbelief, I read the instructions over and over. I thought there must have been a mistake. I took the second test, and once again, two lines quickly appeared. Shock is the only word I could use to describe that moment. I didn't even want to come out of the bathroom because I knew I would have an audience, and I was still trying to digest what was happening. It was such a mix of emotions. I was not trying to have a baby, and I was told I couldn't under the circumstances. On top of all that, Joey and I were seriously struggling in our marriage.

So many things ran through my mind, as I stood staring at myself in that bathroom mirror. I was petrified because my husband and I were having some serious issues that didn't seem to be subsiding. I was worried about money—how could we afford a baby when we could barely pay our mortgage? I jumped months ahead and was ready to cry thinking of dropping my baby off with a caregiver while I worked. I worried about school—how would I finish? I would be disappointing my dad so much (and proving him right). But the biggest fear I had was that my dad would know that I had sex. True story. I was embarrassed knowing that my dad would have confirmation that after three years of marriage, I had sex with my husband. Ridiculous, but true. There's that Italian guilt again!

Walking back to my desk was a blur. Employees not only from my department, but from entirely different floors were staring and asking me if I took the test. I told them, "No," because I didn't want to cause a stir. Instead, I walked directly into my manager's office and looked him dead in the eye. He said with a smirk, "Told ya."

Once I made it back to my desk, still in shock, I called my husband at work. He was still working for the airline with my stepbrother as his crew chief. My stepbrother answered the phone. I said, "Hi, it's me. Can I talk to Joey?"

He responded, "I'll have him call you back in about an hour, he's working a flight."

I said, "I need to talk to him right now, it's very important." He laughed out loud and said, "Very important huh? What? Are you pregnant? We have a flight going off, I can't just pull him off of his post. He will call you back."

I gave a long pause, realizing that was a bit too much of a coincidence to handle in my state, and demanded he figure it out and get him on the phone. His tone changed to serious, and he asked, "Are you ok? What's going on? Jesus, *are* you pregnant?"

I said, "I think so, so I need to talk to him."

He was ecstatic and ran off to get Joey. Joey got on the phone, with his crew members staring at him, and I told him I took a pregnancy test, and it came out positive. He was absolutely shocked. Keep in mind, we weren't trying, we had not suspected anything, and we had not discussed the topic since my diagnosis three years prior.

Still in disbelief, but knowing what I had to do, I made a doctor's appointment. I wasn't going to truly believe it until a doctor told me so. I went to the doctor's appointment alone the next day. I was still thinking there was some kind of mistake, so I took it all very lightly. But things were about to be not so light when the doctor soon confirmed my pregnancy. I called Joey as soon as I left the doctor's office. As it started to sink in and I heard Joey's excitement, I began to get excited too. Joey cries at everything, so he cried, and I tried to cry, but couldn't. I may have still been in disbelief, or it could have been that there were so many times in my life when something good would happen, immediately followed by something bad, so I felt like I was afraid to get too excited.

My due date was unclear due to not knowing when I ovulated last, so after a few weeks and hearing the heartbeat, my doctor sent me in for an ultrasound. Joey and I both went to this appointment. Back then, they would allow a VHS tape so the parents could take it home as a memento. The technician looked at her screen and seemed a bit confused. She looked back and forth through my file and the computer screen. She asked us, "Why are you here today?"

I explained that we were there to confirm the due date because I wasn't sure when I conceived.

She gave a long pause and said seriously, "You have two babies. You do know that, right?"

Joey's knees buckled, but he caught himself right before he hit the ground. If I thought I was in disbelief before, I was in total shock now. We were super excited, crazy happy, and completely out of our minds as we asked her a million questions. We were yelling, "Are you sure? Are you sure?"

She pointed out two heads, and all kinds of other limbs that we could not make heads or tails of. She was sure, and she called the doctor into the room. He confirmed two healthy babies at nineteen weeks. They were kind enough to let us videotape this ultrasound, so having this on tape was the perfect way to tell the grandparents. We drove right to my mom's house first, just telling her we have the video that we wanted her to see, but not telling her we were expecting twins. We popped the tape in and as she watched, the technician had a great shot of both heads. The technician had frozen the screen and typed the numbers 1 and 2 over the heads.

My mom and stepfather were so confused. My mom asked, "What are we looking at? I thought that was a head."

I said, "It is a head."

She asked, "Well then, what is the other thing?"

I said, "Another head!"

She screamed, "Are you having twins?!"

We screamed, and cried, and hugged for what seemed like hours. Then it was off to the other set of parent's homes. It was like we were telling them we were pregnant again, but it seemed ten times more exciting!

This was about the time that Joey took being the provider to the next level. It seemed as if he grew up overnight. And I began to think maybe we had hope after all. He started studying for his real estate license. He passed the test and started selling immediately. He was making enough money to allow me to stay home with our babies if I wanted to. Turns out, that is exactly what I did.

Chapter 11

BABIES ... AND
OTHER HAZARDS OF SEX ...

I started having contractions at twenty-two weeks and was put on bedrest. In my mind, with the constant need to "do something," and then "do some more," I thought bedrest would be the perfect time to get caught up with home projects. A few weeks later at one of my check-ups, my doctor clarified the bed rest rules. He told me he that if I did not start listening to him and stay in bed, he would put me in the hospital. He explained the survival rate of babies born at this gestational period. And he scared me to my core.

For the next two and a half months, I was only allowed to lay down or sit with my feet elevated. This was pre-internet, so I watched TV with my credit card and phone next to me. I ordered the entire 70s hits on CDs over time. I also read Twin books and of course, the bible for expectant mothers, "What to Expect When You're Expecting."

In the meantime, Joey took this time to "rest" himself. I begged him to get the nursery set up and do the million other things that needed to be done before we took two babies home from the hospital in a few weeks. And in my unending determination that I could handle it all, I tried to do it myself. He procrastinated with everything, and I was forced to lay in bed all day, losing my mind knowing the nursery wasn't ready for our sweet babies. I was in what you call the nesting phase—I *needed* a nest!

I threw a fit. I got up and tried to get the crib mattresses and cribs down from a high shelf in the garage myself. In retrospect, I realize what a bad decision that was. I realize the consequences could have been catastrophic. To this day, I lose sleep over that and not sure I will ever forgive myself for taking that risk. I should have asked for help from my mom or anyone, but I was also pretending everything was still great. I was also hiding the fact that Joey was out after work and would never do anything to help me in the house.

I was miserable those last few months. I had had a migraine headache exactly every other day for the entire duration of my pregnancy. I was so nauseous I was barely eating and at times, could barely get water down. I was in the ER five times during these last months hooked up to an IV to try to stop the contractions.

Then, at thirty-three weeks, I delivered two baby girls! By the grace of God, they were breathing on their own, but the next few days were extremely scary. They were 4.9 pounds and 5.1 pounds, jaundiced, and could not regulate their body temperatures on their own. They were under heat lamps, and all bundled up with two onesies, two coddling blankets, another very big blanket, and hats.

When they let me take them home a few days later, I was so scared. They were so tiny. While I had a ton of nieces and nephews and had changed their diapers, fed them, and given them baths, I never had to care for a baby full time, and certainly not two, both of whom needed extra special care. I never felt the heavy weight of responsibility as I had in that moment. These two precious babies were counting on me. And I was in my early twenties and felt utterly alone, with a husband who seemed more like a child himself than the other person who should have shared this responsibility with me.

When the heavy weight of all that I had before me would subside, I would be in awe. These babies were my whole world. I couldn't even look at them without crying. I had no idea how, in this lifetime, I became so lucky! I would rather sit and stare at them than do anything else in the world. My friends were out and about being twenty-four-year-olds—clubbing, meeting guys, taking boat trips on Lake Michigan, and living it up. But I didn't feel like I was missing a thing. I was perfectly happy where I was.

I was also extremely protective of my girls. I had this constant fear that something terrible might happen to one of them. Remembering my own childhood, I promised them I would always use good judgment on every decision concerning them, or myself. I promised them that they would always come first—no matter what.

The next several months were very tough for me. Postpartum depression set in. I also wasn't able to produce enough milk to breastfeed both babies. And after many tears and many sleepless nights, worrying they weren't getting enough, I took my doctor's advice to stop. This had an unintended impact of making me feel like a total failure—I couldn't even feed my babies. Would I really be able to protect them? I was at my mom's house almost every weekend for her to help me, but during the week, she was busy working.

Joey's second career in real estate was taking a lot of his time, but he was determined to make it work, so that I could stay home with our babies. I truly appreciated that, but it also meant he was never home to help and never home for me in general. When he saw that I was struggling, he sent his mom in his place. She loved helping me and loved being with the girls so much.

She would drop everything, even leave work without pay, to drive an hour to get to me any time she was asked. She would do it even if she wasn't asked. She would insist on coming over so I could have a break.

She would insist on staying over and get up with them in the middle of the night. *Amazing, right?*

My problem was that I had this uncontrollable, unjustified fear something bad would happen to them if I wasn't the one taking care of them. I was afraid no one could do it like it needed to be done. I was scared maybe someone else might be careless because no one could possibly love them like I did. Ultimately, I was scared God would take them from me because I didn't believe I deserved them in the first place. I am not sure why, but I tend to think it had to do with my insecurities growing up and being treated the way I was treated. But, regardless of all those feelings, my mother-in-law was Godsent at that time.

I also think I harbored some misplaced resentment toward her because I thought my husband should be the one doing this with me. I wanted a partner. I wanted a family unit, with him as the dad, doing dad things, and us experiencing this great gift together. But that seemed as if it would never happen. I thought if she wouldn't have been there, maybe he would. Looking back, I know I didn't appreciate her for the efforts she was making because of this. If I could change one thing about this time in my life, I would have appreciated her more. I wish I knew then what I know now. I wish I appreciated her help more. If I had the opportunity, I would thank her wholeheartedly for all her love and dedication to her granddaughters, and to me.

Through all the tears and all the resentment and sleepless nights, I did appreciate my husband's hard work. I will always be grateful to him for his work ethic to take care of his family financially. If he had not taken on the burden of two full-time jobs, I would have never had the opportunity to stay home to take care of our babies. The real problem came in when that pressure of being the sole provider began to take a toll on him. To cope, he started rewarding himself for a job well done. In the little time he had, he started going out with his friends even more, rather than coming home to be with his family. I don't have one recollection of him being home after work to spend time with us or to help me. The first memory I have of us as a family was the following summer when I would bring our one-year-olds to his softball games. If he wouldn't come to us, we would go to him. *I guess that would have to be okay.*

Chapter 12

A BABY, A BOBCAT, AND BAMBI

When the twins were two years old, I became pregnant again. I was ovulating more regularly, so we probably should have been more careful if we weren't ready for a third baby. To be honest, I never even wanted to have sex with him because I was so disgusted by his lack of familial engagement, so I don't even know how I got pregnant.

I was not sorry though. I knew we could make it work. I was already home with the girls, and he had his work schedule. Having all my babies so close in age was ideal in my mind. I wanted them all to be close. Remembering the beginning with the twins, I was a little scared of the work involved. All those worries, and some new ones, came flooding back. I was scared wondering if I could love another baby like I did my twins. But I also remembered that loving my twins the way I did showed me that I have so much love to give. We would be okay.

When we went for the ultrasound for this pregnancy, I was actually hoping for twins again. Having twins was more rewarding than it was work, and I absolutely loved every day with my girls. The ultrasound showed one baby—one healthy baby—and I was extremely grateful. During the pregnancy, everyone was asking, "Are you hoping for a boy now that you have two girls?"

My answer, "To be honest, I just want a healthy baby, but if I had to make a choice, I'd choose to have another girl."

Knowing we were going to outgrow our small townhouse in no time, we decided it was time to get into something bigger. I was extremely reluctant, as I knew it would only mean more work for me. Joey still did nothing to help me at all, ever. Not the girls, not the housework, not the cooking, not the laundry. Nothing. He swore once he had his own house, it would be different. I didn't believe him. He was still working two full-time jobs and rewarding himself by going out with his friends, drinking, or playing softball or golf, whenever he wasn't working.

To make the finances work out to get a construction loan for the property we purchased, the bank needed us to get our debt to income right. To do so, we had to sell our townhouse. My amazing sister took us in during this time. She only had one spare bedroom, so we had a twin bed set up, and two cribs and a dresser. The cribs were rail to rail so the twins would often climb over in the middle of the night and sleep together—scary, but adorable to see them cuddled so close. This was a big adjustment for us all, but somehow, we made it work.

I was also pregnant at the time—never a fun time to not be in your own room or even bed. We were hoping our house to be done before the delivery, but we were not even close. We broke ground on our home just one week before our new baby was born. Not good timing, but we were at the mercy of dealing with approvals from the county, as we bought a piece of property in an unincorporated area. Fortunately, my father-in-law was a handyman and ended up being in charge of many of the jobs we needed.

Just before I delivered our baby, we got an apartment. There was no way we could fit another crib, or even a small bassinet into the bedroom of my sister's house. But none of that mattered when I saw that God blessed me with another baby girl! And one thing was for sure, I wanted to name my baby after my dad, Joe.

Sometimes, when you are in the midst of chaos—in this case, raising three girls all under the age of three—you don't notice when someone very close to you is spiraling out of control. But I had remembered it clearly with my dad years before when he was managing my out-of-control sister, his elderly mother with dementia, and my stepmom with her drinking addiction. This time, my husband was the one circling the drain and threatening to take our beautiful family along with him. These things are difficult to notice when you're in the moment though.

After our precious baby girl was born, completing our family, Joey's behavior only got worse—he started staying out all night and took on a new travel softball league. He would continue to travel with his buddies for three-to-four-day weekends in Vegas, or golf trips around the country. He was having the time of his life (at least on the surface), while I was becoming more and more lonely and depressed.

It was so incredibly difficult to see him self-destruct, seemingly in slow motion. He turned into someone I no longer knew (and to be honest, didn't like very much) and it became unbearable. I often asked him, "How can you think it is ok for you to be putting dollars into a stripper's thong, while I'm home clipping coupons to try to put enough food on the table?" He never answered. He did tell me I should get a hobby though. That was his answer.

I remember that when I would open up to some friends, I would always be asked, "Why do you let him get away with doing these things?" As if I was *allowing* it. As if I had any choice in the matter. To be clear, Joey, much like my stepfather and stepbrothers did while I was growing up, did whatever he wanted to do. Fun with the fellas always seemed to trump time with his growing family. And consequences be damned!

I did convince him to go to marriage counseling with me. I wanted this to work. I remembered how in love we used to be. We had a family now, but I knew myself enough to know I would not live the rest of my life like this. And within that short hour of us sitting with this stranger, I knew I was going to divorce him. He spent that time not being concerned with how I felt or how to make our marriage work, but instead negotiating how many times a week was *fair* for him to go out with his friends. This was a married man with three babies at home, and all he could think about was how much time could he spend *away* from us.

About three months into building the new house, my father-in-law got a small taste of what I was dealing with for years. I could tell he was at his wits end by the way he ignored Joey at the family Christmas party, except to tell him that he quit. He had every right to wonder how he could be the only one working while he saw his son each day with too much of a hangover to even remotely pitch in. So, he left. He had that option. He simply stepped off the job and left our soon-to-be house without a roof and only the first floor of plywood down … in the middle of the winter. Much like our faltering family, our house was hanging on by a thread (or piece of plywood).

I couldn't really blame him though. If anyone knew how he felt, I did. When Joey did show up to work on the house, he would often be sent to the hardware store for parts. *Great—do something!* But when he would go to the "store," he would usually be gone for hours at a time. *Hey, how can you really pass a pub when a game is on and not stop, right?* So, all the workers at the house would be standing around waiting for the supplies that were sitting in his backseat, while he was drinking at one bar or another with his buddies.

Disappointed is the understatement of the world. Not only did I have three babies in a small apartment, waiting for our home to be built (which seemed impossible most days), but I was watching the man who had really been my best friend destroy his life. He was such a good guy, a family guy, who was so good with his nieces and nephews. I had thought for sure I was going to have the best dad for my kids. I just could not reconcile these two people. I could not understand what had happened to the man I loved.

The stand-off with my father-in-law went on for about two months. Finally, he must have realized that he was not going to be able to teach his son a lesson at this stage in his life. He could see that his daughter-in-law was struggling to take care of his three granddaughters alone in an extremely cramped two-bedroom apartment. For us, he started working again. A few months later, we were issued a "temporary" occupancy permit. I thought I would cry I was so happy and relieved.

There were several items that still needed to be completed before the final permit was issued— land grading and the septic field, to name a few. I'm not sure what made me think I was going to get help with these things, but by this time, we ran out of money completely and had to do the work we could by ourselves. Grading dirt? Piece of cake. We just had to have several yards of dirt dumped and rent a Bobcat to spread it. I didn't care. I needed my house done! The Bobcat was delivered, but Joey let it sit too long. Then, it was time for the Bobcat to go back and we didn't have any more money to rent it again. And even if we did, I knew the chances of him actually doing something with it were slim to none.

As a consequence, he would have to spread yards of dirt by hand. But Joey never did anything he didn't want to do. Ever. He found time to go out with his friends and generally make every effort to not come home at night. But when faced with the challenge of making sure his family's home was safe and sound, he just couldn't be bothered.

It was going to be left up to me. I knew if we didn't get this done, we would lose our occupancy permit. And homeless with three toddlers is not a good look … for anyone. The final inspection was right around the corner, so, once again, I did what I had to do. I had to spread yards of dirt by myself. I had a shovel, a wheel barrel, and a rake, with three babies in tow. And meanwhile, from what I could tell he was stuffing that Bobcat money in Bambi's thong at the Gold Club.

The inspection only went well because the inspectors felt so sorry for me. This is not a normal emotion for most inspectors. The grading was not to their standard. How could it be? I had very little to work with. They passed it with the promise that we would fix what needed to be fixed as soon as possible. Of course, that never happened, and we had floods often. But I had my girls in their home.

Chapter 13

CHRISTMAS EVE

In the insanity that was our house being built, Joey had an idea. He thought my maternal grandmother should move in with us. He said we would have an apartment built in the basement (not that he would do it, of course). My mother and her siblings thought this would be a great idea, too. My cousins and sisters all promised they'd help. But I didn't feel as confident as everyone else. I knew I would be alone, taking care of another responsibility. And I already felt like I was at a breaking point. How much more did they all want from me?

Still, I thought—*Okay, as long as everyone will pitch in when I need them, I can do this.* The consensus was that she would help me with the kids, so it would be a great trade off. But, as I expected, that trade off never happened. My grandmother was very demanding from day one. We had a clear role reversal transpiring. Having her there was like having another child, except I couldn't put her in a time out. After about three months of this behavior, she was diagnosed with a malignant brain tumor, so her behavior started to make sense. She had brain surgery, but Grandma never went back to being herself. She was demanding and childish. And I became resentful as my mom and sisters couldn't make it during the week or at least on a regular basis to pitch in. And all those cousins who were going to help, only showed up one time—and all on the same day.

This time in my life was probably the most challenging up to that point, even harder than my childhood. I had so many people counting on me in so many ways. I was being a mommy to three little girls, taking care of my elderly grandmother, trying to manage my husband's drinking, gambling, and time away from home, all while I took on babysitting full time for three other small children, under the age of four, just to make ends meet. I was overwhelmed, bitter, and felt completely taken advantage of from so many.

Honestly, I don't even know how I was able to put a smile on my face for my kids. I had to remind myself daily that this was not their fault and that I was not going to take any of this out on them. I actually think I did a pretty good job not letting them know the stress I was under. They don't seem to have any recollection of this hectic time.

Of course, there was also the incredible loneliness and uncertainty. I never knew if Joey was going to come home at night. I never knew if the parents of these children I was babysitting for were going to pick up their kids on time. I never knew if my grandmother was going to wake up in a good mood or a bad mood. All I wanted was to spend time with my kids without being interrupted with everyone else's bullshit. I cannot remember two days connecting that wasn't interrupted with someone interfering with my life.

Just a few months after my grandmother's brain surgery and only six months after we moved into our home, on December 6, 1998, my father went into the ER with spells of passing out. All the doctors had to do was figure out that his heart meds and blood pressure meds needed to be regulated. But somehow, during his stay, he became even more ill. We now know that on the day he was admitted he contracted a staph infection—a staph infection that would take his life only eighteen days later, on Christmas Eve.

The nurses and doctors told us day after day that he was going to be released at any time. But we saw the staff neglect him, while carrying on with their holiday celebrations at their nurse's stations. It was disgusting. There were also too many doctors involved with his diagnoses, as if there were too many cooks in the kitchen. No one knew what was going on. And the only commonalty they had was that they were non-attentive.

The frustration for us as a family was unbearable. It was also a very strange time for those of us closest to him. My sister, who in my eyes, had tortured him most of her life, came out of nowhere like "Daughter of the Year," and spent every chance she had at his bedside. We weren't sure what her motive was—there was always an ulterior motive. We all stood around watching, scratching our heads, knowing whatever her reason was underneath all the niceties, her presence was likely good for our dad. I thought (and hoped) for a split second that maybe she changed and turned into an empathetic human being. I was wrong.

On the afternoon of December 24th, we were all called to the hospital in a hurry. My aunt called me on the phone, "We are on our way to the hospital. Something went terribly wrong, and we all need to get there as soon as we can."

I was just cleaning up from having my in-laws over for Christmas Eve breakfast and getting ready to go to my mom's house, where she hosts about fifty of us every year. Joey told me to go and that he would take care of the kids and meet me at my mom's. I briefly thought it was a Christmas miracle for him to help with his own kids, but I didn't have more than a second to give him my thoughts. My only concern was my dad. I jumped in my car and noticed halfway to the hospital that, of course, was *somehow* left on empty. I wouldn't make it. I had to stop for gas. At 2:02 p.m. as I pulled up at the gas station, still fifteen minutes from the hospital, I heard my dad's voice in my head, "Awe, Lin." He hated that I drove without a full tank of gas at all times.

When I arrived, I walked into his hospital room. He was just lying there. I thought he was asleep, but then I noticed all of the machines in the room were off. There was no annoying beeping sounds (that I would have loved to hear in that moment), no lights blinking as if in Morse Code, no numbers flashing on tiny screens. The bed sheets were neat, and they were pulled up to mid chest. A male nurse came in and said, "Oh, you shouldn't be in here. Let me bring you to your family."

I said, "But he's my dad..."

He didn't respond. I said it again, and he walked me to a room, opened the door, where my not-so-nice sister was sitting next to my stepmom. I looked at my sister's face and was still confused. I was in denial. She started crying, and shaking her head, and I asked her, "WHAT? Did he die? Is he dead?"

She nodded yes and grabbed me and tried to hug me. I immediately started crying and gagging, and my stepmom quickly grabbed the garbage can and held it under my mouth. There are no words to describe the feeling when you find out that your parent has died. It means forever. They are not coming back. Ever. I felt as if my entire world was pulled away from me and I was floating somewhere in space, with nothing to tie me down. All of my security, all of my faith was gone in that instance. At 2:02pm, he was pronounced dead. That was the exact time I looked at my clock in my car and heard his voice talk to me.

With the passing of my dad, my rock, I thought my life was over. I am shocked that I was able to go on with my everyday life. I didn't think I could. I didn't think I was strong enough. I know my dad would have been disappointed in me if I just gave up and shut down. That gave me incentive to get out of bed the next day. My little girls needed me to still be a good mommy. They were counting on me. I needed to be strong and know our lives had to go on.

Looking back, I have no idea how I survived this along with all the other obstacles going on at once, none of which I had control over. But I guess, as a survivor, I knew nothing else but to put one foot in front of the other and move forward. After all, what else can we do?

I know if it weren't for my kids I would have wanted to give up. There were just so many things out of my control directly affecting me in such negative ways. I could not control my husband's drinking. I could not control my husband's gambling and lack of interest in his family. I could not control my grandmother's behavior. I could not control my father's death. And then, just when I thought it couldn't get any worse, my life was physically threatened because my husband couldn't break up with his bookie.

Chapter 14

THE THREAT

The phone ring late one night. Joey, of course, wasn't home. I, of course, was taking care of our sick one-and-a-half year old with a fever alone.

"Hello," I answered, bouncing her on my hip to try to get her to stop crying.

"Hey Linda. It's Tony." Tony was a "friend" of Joey's at the time.

"Hi Tony. What's going on?"

"I'm calling to see if you sent me the check yet," he answered.

"Check for what?" *Seriously, I don't need this shit right now.*

"Joey owes me $500 for last week."

"Well, I guess you'll have to talk to Joey then. I don't know anything about it."

"Well, you do now. You need to get that money to me. It needs to be in the mail. Today."

"Tony, I cannot leave the house. My daughter is sick and throwing up. And, like I said, this is not between you and me. This is Joey's issue."

"Not anymore it isn't. See, I'm not asking you. I'm telling you what you are going to do. You will get what is coming, not Joey."

I slammed the phone down, thinking—*Did that mother fucker just threaten my life? And did my husband actually put my life at risk?*

We had just refinanced our house and rolled $40,000 into the mortgage to clear up our credit cards. Some of the debt was last minute house expenses, but most of it was subsidizing Joey's personal life choices. And now, we needed to pay off his gambling debt or face … God only knows.

I asked myself how many more times I was willing to do this and let him drag us down financially. How much more debt was I willing to take on because of him? I had three little girls to take care of. Three little girls, who had *real* needs and would soon have a lot more—and many of them would cost money. There would be sports or dance lessons, tutors, and extracurricular activities. There would be more clothes, shoes, and food. Plus, I needed some damn stability in my life. I didn't want to live like this anymore. Why couldn't he see what he was doing to me? To our family? Why didn't he care enough to do something about it?

I couldn't help but wonder, if we lost our home, what would happen to my girls? I had not yet finished my undergraduate degree, so even if I were to get a full-time job, it would be minimum pay. How could I support them? I wouldn't even be able to support myself at minimum wage. Feelings of inadequacy and being stuck in a helpless situation resurfaced from my childhood. And once again, I felt alone

When Joey came home, I threatened him with divorce. It did not faze him. He laughed in my face and said, "Who is going to want you with three kids?"

Sadly, I believed him. So, I decided to make one more attempt to save my failing marriage. One of my dearest friends and her husband had come over for an intervention with us and suggested that we go to this magical weekend. I asked him to go on this marriage retreat, and he agreed. He always *did* like to travel.

My friend who recommended the retreat said it would change our lives. And she was right. It changed our lives for the better indeed … temporarily.

Chapter 15

PAIN MORPHS INTO A PLAN

With the help of a counselor at the retreat, we came up with a fair number of days a week he was "allowed" to go out after work. And he stuck to it. I saw the difference in our financials immediately. He wasn't spending as much money on his personal hobbies, like drinking, playing softball, traveling with the boys, and golf, which made it much easier for me to pay the bills … and on time. In return, I agreed to a clean slate with no grudges. Soon, I started trusting him again and amazingly, fell in love all over again. I was able to get intimate with him more regularly. Something that I had absolutely no interest in previously, after the way he was behaving prior to counseling.

My aunt in Florida reluctantly took my grandmother in to save me some stress, and I knew I had to start creating some positive energy in my life. Things started looking up. I actually began to feel like I had gotten some control back in my life. I was able to put some order and stability back into our marriage and family. My mind, thoughts, emotions, and overall state of being were all headed in a positive direction. This tends to happen when you get rid of toxic situations.

Joey gave up real estate and started working at a golf course. Over the years, his golfing adventures led to some great connections, and through one of them, he found an opportunity to head the caddy program at a well-known golf course. He loved this job! Working somewhere that he loved brought him to a good place mentally. It gave him less hours at a job that put too many temptations to go out drinking every night, and more hours with members of a country club, where he seemingly wanted to be on his best behavior. He was so well respected at this club that he was recommended for a more prestigious job at another club.

Things were looking up, all around. He was doing great. The girls were thriving. Our bills were being paid. I felt better and more in control of our lives. I finally had a sense of peace that I hadn't had in a long time (if ever). But, as we all know, when we think we've figured it out most is when life shows us that we know absolutely nothing.

Less than six months into this new job, just when I thought our marriage was back where it belonged, Joey stayed late after work one night … and then another … and then some more. I quickly saw the writing on the wall and just couldn't believe it. He was spending less time at home, and once again, I lost all trust and faith in him. I knew at that moment that I had done all that I could over the years to save us, but as they say, it takes two to do such things. I was the only one I could truly count on—some things never change.

One night, thinking these thoughts over and over again, feeling myself slip into the old negative thoughts and patterns, I remembered my control. So, I decided to make a five-year plan. I knew well enough that change does not happen overnight. I knew I needed time and I needed to work toward my goals—that's what this plan was for me. It was a way to get the control back that I was losing a little more each and every day with Joey. I had yet one more toxic situation to get out of.

That night, I wrote it all down:

My Five-Year Plan …

Back to college. Finish up my undergraduate degree, so I can get a job that pays enough to support my three little ones and myself.

Get my little one settled into 1ˢᵗ grade, so there is minimal day care.

Start my journey of getting my body into better shape. Someone will be seeing me naked again at some point again.

Begin the process of eating healthy foods again and incorporate some of my nutrition knowledge into my life so I could feel good and make clear headed decisions.

Begin to adjust to the idea of selling my home and moving into a small apartment that I could afford on my own.

With a plan in place, I felt better immediately. But I also needed money now. So, I decided rather than make minimum wage somewhere, I would start my own business, giving me money and flexibility. I was always pretty creative and liked putting things together. I don't remember exactly how it all clicked into place, but I decided I would use these skills in a gift basket business. And I was good at it. I grew the business without the help of the internet to several clients through word of mouth and self-promotion. My aunt was kind enough to get me in front of the Marshall Field's Travel department. The executive there gave me the incredible opportunity to service their high clientele. I also picked up another client who serviced the Board of Trade in Chicago. There were several more clients who kept me busy enough that I was able to have something of my own that I felt really good about. I had created something, and it was proving fruitful, not only monetarily, but for my own emotional and mental well-being.

My mom helped me at trade shows and my sisters (yes sisters, even the one who made me feel like she hated me) came in to help spend time with my kids during deliveries and sometimes help me make bows for the basket toppers. My stepmom gave me a loan to get a jump start with inventory, my mother-in-law and Joey's aunt helped me with the kids. I knew I had had a support system before, but WOW! They really came to support me at this time, and I was so grateful. There's no feeling in the world like feeling like you have people in your corner. People who love you and want nothing more than to see you succeed. There were many times in my life I didn't feel that, but other times, like then, that it blew me away.

I received the most amazing, positive feedback from clients and the recipients of the gift baskets that it fueled my passion to do even more—to do even better. I was earning an income to cover the loss from Joey's bad habits, and I had a positive outlook. I felt like I was teaching my kids some great work ethics, even at their very young ages. It was important to me that they saw their mommy working. I don't think they considered my babysitting or my teaching CCD (Catholic Communion classes) or my coaching soccer as "real jobs" (I actually volunteered at the latter two, so the girls could attend for free because I couldn't afford to send them), so now they saw that not only did I have a real job, I had my own business!

The business generated enough revenue for me to buy a nice car for my basket deliveries. I could not show up in the beater minivan that we bought for $1,000 back when we needed more room. It was extremely embarrassing and would not look right pulling up to the Board of Trade or Marshall Field's with gift baskets that were likely worth more than the van itself. And any extra money I made allowed us to get some credit card and gambling debt paid. But we were so far in the dark debt hole, my commendable attempts barely made a dent.

My business could have, and would have, skyrocketed if I had the time, and resources to learn more about sales on the internet. In the late 1990s and early 2000s, it was really just getting going and I had no idea where to start. I just couldn't do it, and I had no one to help me in that respect. I did okay working through my FAX machine, but looking back, I wish I would have pursued the right help at that time. I had the family help for the personal side of things, but I did not have the right people to help on the business side. At the time, I didn't appreciate what a truly exceptional achievement this had been. I had built something from absolutely nothing.

About two years later and surviving three Christmas orders and deliveries for the business, I had another life decision to make. We had now lived in our home for about three years, and we had just refinanced for the second time, rolling tens of thousands more into our mortgage. We were fortunate that our home had appreciated a great deal, leaving us room to do this because there was no convincing Joey to change his ways.

My business kept me busy enough that I had little time left to pay attention to Joey's behavior. He was working a lot, I was working a lot, and I started caring less and less if he came home or not. Based on the blatant immature behavior and the disrespect that he was displaying, it seemed as though he was starting to resent me for doing something to keep myself in a positive place. *Huge red flag there! As if I needed another.*

If and when we would have dinner as a family, he would start acting out by farting at the dinner table or burping in my face. If I asked him to pass the buns, and he would throw one at me. The kids thought he was funny. I found it disgusting and disrespectful. It was as if I had four children at the dinner table. In fact, our daughters, as young as they were, acted with more manners. He had never done anything like this before. I had to explain to him I was trying to raise little ladies, but he just didn't care. He would undermine me in front of them. If I was upstairs, and the phone rang and it was for me, he would whistle at me like I was a dog to tell me I had a phone call.

I would take the kids to church every Sunday. One Sunday when he happened to be home, he asked where we were going. I told him that I take the kids to church every Sunday and asked if he wanted to go. He said, "No, I'm not going. Why do they have to go every Sunday? We don't have to go."

The kids looked at me expectantly and said, "Yeah, we don't want to go."

Suddenly, with his one thoughtless comment, they thought it was now optional. It wasn't to me. Every week from that Sunday on, the kids gave me push back about going to church. I felt that the more I put myself first, gaining control of the structure of the household and started making a life for myself, the more he regressed. And worst of all, this disrespectful behavior reminded me of how my stepdad and stepbrothers used to treat me. It was so in your face that I was appalled by it, reliving the past horror of my childhood. It was time to execute my plan.

Chapter 16

A NEW START

In the Winter of 2000, I enrolled at DePaul University. When I was put on bedrest with my first pregnancy, I had to drop the classes in which I had been enrolled. I didn't have many more classes to take, but this was a different college and a different time, so wasn't sure what to expect. There was an adult program that was perfect for me, and I was able to use a majority of my previous classes as credits. I was on track to earn my undergraduate degree at a part-time pace in three years.

Once again, my amazing friends and family came to my aid to help babysit my kids, so I could attend school. My sisters (yes, both of them), one of my best friends, my mom, mother-in-law, and Joey's aunt helped make my educational pursuit happen. And I can never thank them enough for that because Joey was no help or support whatsoever.

Unfortunately, Joey's behavior continued. He would tell me he would be home for dinner, then not come home until after the kids were in bed. No phone calls. No explanations. He would take a day off work, and I would foolishly get excited thinking we would be doing a family thing, only to find out that he made plans to go golfing instead. Those "golf days" would last from 6:00 a.m. until midnight, so we wouldn't see him at all. I asked him once to help me paint the living room. He only would agree to it if I would agree to let him go to Vegas with the boys for four days. This was my life—constant deals and negotiations to get more time away from us. That is also when he was paying for these trips for all his friends. Car rentals and hotel stays would go on our credit cards, with the promise they would pay us back. Of course, they never did (or if they did, the money went right into Joey's pockets).

School gave me another outlet. Similar to the business, it gave me another way to set my mind on a positive path—another way to remind myself that I could do anything I set my mind to, which I now call, "Words of Affirmation." All these positives gave me reason to wake up in a good mood every day. I missed my dad like crazy, but I became even closer to my mom during this time. She became my head cheerleader, taking the role my dad had been in my entire life. Looking back, she was always in my corner, but because my father was the captain of the cheer squad, I don't think I paid enough attention to all that my mom did for me over the years. It was being overshadowed by her role with my stepfather for so long.

Along with starting classes, I started a workout program. I wanted to get myself into shape. To be honest, I had no idea what I was doing. I did a ton of cardio because I could hit "quick start," on the treadmill, and thought that was what I needed—a quick start! I cut my calories down to almost nothing. I was eating my kids leftover French toast squares right off their plates, the crusts off their peanut butter and jelly sandwiches, and then I would usually sit with them with a plate of meat and pasta at dinner time.

I don't recall ever making myself plates of food for breakfast or lunch ever since my kids were born. I only remember eating while standing up and running around serving everyone else. So, my caloric intake was always low, but in addition to the low calories, I increased my cardiovascular activity. This program that I thought I had mastered to get to my fitness goal actually did all the wrong things to me. I caused my body to steal nutrients from my muscle, lowering my metabolism, and then caused my body to burn off muscle by overdoing cardio. Initially I started getting smaller, but then gained fat as a result. Still, it's all about the lessons learned.

In the meantime, it became very clear that Joey resented me when he saw me taking charge of my life. Maybe he was finally starting to feel threatened? After all, I had warned him, and even though he thought I'd never do it, he likely wondered what he would do without me. He did very little to take care of himself or our home. I did all the cooking, cleaning, and laundry. I made lunches (including his), I took care of the kids, and all the household chores, including mowing the lawn and taking out the garbage. I think he may have started getting scared that I might actually follow through with my threat.

And I did. To me, it wasn't a threat. It was reality. I told him I was not going to live my life like this. And I wasn't. It wasn't a fast, clean break, *and* the series of events that pushed it along were a bit controversial, but eventually, I did it.

Chapter 17

TAKING CARE OF MYSELF ... FOR ONCE

One day, I was in a large common area while I was in between classes. A bunch of people came out of a classroom, circling around who I assumed to be a guest speaker in the class. This man, I found out later, was there lecturing on terrorism, but they were now talking about working out, getting fit, and how to get the body into the perfect balance, so it would lose weight and be efficient. I couldn't help but eavesdrop, as these were the issues I had been struggling with recently.

Someone noticed me getting into the conversation, and they gave me an opening to ask a question. I found out during the next five minutes that whatever I was doing to get myself into shape was the exact opposite of what I should be doing! Before the conversation was over, this group invited me to be part of their workout group and to meet them on a regular basis at a local gym. Talk about the right place at the right time. Not only was I going to get some great, free advice, but I would get together with a group of people with the same goals and outlook on health, and life. I was thrilled.

Not long after, I was attending one of my classes on a Sunday afternoon, while my mother-in-law was watching my girls. She dropped me off at class and then was going to pick me up after—we only had the one car. The campus was a ghost town on Sundays, so there were very few cars in the parking lot. I walked out of the building and walked into the parking lot when I did not see her up front. I stood there waiting for about twenty minutes.

At that time, the Master Trainer, Nate (the lecturer I had met the other day) walked out of the building and saw me standing there alone. He asked what was going on and I told him I was waiting for my ride. He insisted on waiting with me. He said, "I cannot drive away leaving you alone, standing in this parking lot."

I tried calling my mother-in-law several times, but she didn't answer. After about twenty more minutes of standing there having small talk with a man who I had only met a handful of times, he asked if I would like to sit in his car or if I thought it would look bad if my mother-in-law drove up on that. Well, all I knew was that I was tired of standing for the last forty minutes, so I told him sure. During this alone time in his car, we discussed a workout plan for me, and I committed to a couple of days of workouts during the week. We were able to work out a schedule, so I could have designated days and times to train. It was the only way I could do it, with having to coordinate time for babysitters. Getting in shape was part of my five-year-plan, and I was determined to see it all through. I had let myself go, not only mentally and emotionally, but also physically over the past eight years.

Within a few minutes in the car, of course, my mother-in-law drove up, quickly ending our brief conversation. I introduced her to Nate and thanked him for waiting with me, so I wouldn't be alone and finally had a place to sit, instead of standing in the middle of the parking lot. She apologized and said she lost track of time. And that was the end of that … or so I thought.

I started meeting Nate and his friends at the gym, which eventually dwindled down to just meeting him. It turned out that he was a Master Trainer for the United States Government—not a bad title. He really seemed to know what he was doing, and was probably the smartest, most patient person I had ever met. He was a lot like my dad, in fact! I really needed people in my life who would help keep me on track and accountable to myself, so this was great!

It seemed that the better I was starting to feel outside the home, the worse I felt inside it, though. Joey started making things very difficult for me to get away to go to classes and especially the gym. I had to start counting on friends and family members once again. This is also about the time when he started calling me "selfish" because clearly taking time away from my kids to workout was "selfish." Talk about irony at its finest. It's apparently not selfish to spend hours and even days away from your kids to go on trips, play golf and softball, and go out drinking, but working out—Oh my God! The audacity I had! Seriously, it was ridiculous!

Joey would say anything to get to me—not horrible things, but things that would work my guilt to no end. He knew I hated leaving my kids for any length of time and I also hated asking people to help. He knew I felt like a burden, and I hated that. But I couldn't stop thinking how insanely ironic it was to accuse ME of being selfish by being away from my kids. Where was he stepping up to fill the void while I took an extra hour here and there for my mental and physical health.

Several weeks into my workout regimen, Joey seemed to become suspicious of my leaving the house, rushing around to coordinate babysitters at specific times, and he started talking to people about it. My mother-in-law heard his concern and mentioned the day weeks earlier that she came to pick me up from school and I was sitting in this man's car. She remembered his name and told Joey.

I believe my in-laws were very aware of what was going on inside our four walls, but they hoped, of course, it would improve. Or they hoped I'd just accept him for who he was, which was not happening. When she told Joey about that day, he called me from work and asked me very firmly, "WHO IS Nate?" I told him the truth right away—I had nothing to hide. He was a guy I met at school that I started working out with.

Before I knew it, I was getting phone calls from friends and family members, asking me how I could cheat on poor Joey. *What?* Somehow, although I think I know how, everyone believed I was cheating, and they were all trying to talk sense into me. Of course, nobody knew what was actually going on in my household. They all thought things were perfect and we were the perfect family! My stepbrothers thought his actions were normal because, well it was normal … to them. And not one of them had any idea of the kind of financial debt and burden we were now dealing with. So, my "bad behavior" (which again, was going to school and working out) was not warranted as far as they were concerned.

I was furious. After all I had done to hold our family, our marriage, and our household together, against all odds, this was the thanks I got—from everyone. Against all the obstacles Joey threw my way. I was so frustrated. The idea that I would try to put myself first for once and try to take care of my mental and physical health, while I had the kids at a sitter caused everyone to think I was crazy, is just that … crazy. I realized that if I wasn't going to start taking care of myself, I wasn't going to be as valuable to my kids as I needed to be. I realized that the stress was eventually going to catch up with me. Once I went to school and met other adults with husbands and wives and listened to the dynamics of their households, I saw that mine was completely upside down. I also saw that I was the only one who could fix it, but I had to be focused and think straight.

What was even more shocking to me was that Joey, at age thirty-two, still behaved, in essence, like a frat boy all this time and nobody judged him. Everyone just shrugged it off—*Oh, you know Joey!* But when I took the time to do something to better my health, they all viewed it as me becoming selfish, a bad mom, and a bad wife. Double standard doesn't even begin to describe it. And it was exactly this double standard that

I was no longer going to tolerate. My mom, being used to "bros being bros," felt like I was overreacting … until I told her about the chaos he was causing. She said, "Wow, I divorced your father for less reason than that!" My sister hated to see a divorce, but she was extremely loyal to me and trusted my judgment. She would do anything to support my happiness.

Back at home though, my daughters now started to act out toward me. I attributed it to learned behavior—their dad was doing it, so why shouldn't they? He was effectively showing them it was okay to treat me that way. But one morning, they noticed him coming home at 7:30 a.m., while they were sitting at the breakfast table. One of them asked, "Daddy, are you just getting home from when you went out last night?"

He had the audacity to accuse me of telling them he stayed out all night. They were eight and five and a half! They knew exactly what was going on. I never told them anything bad that he was doing. I would have done everything to save them those terrible thoughts. On the other hand, his immaturity wouldn't allow him to see that he created this mess—not me.

Chapter 18

A NEW FRIEND

Nate did several things for me while I trained with him. He not only educated me on health and fitness, but he gave me the confidence that was stripped from me ever since I was a child. If there is one lesson for which I could give him credit, it was the phrase he would tell me over and over, "You are a person first, a woman second, and a mother third. If you don't take care of the person you are, you can't possibly be the best mom you can be." Now that made sense. That I could understand. That I could get behind. That helped take away the guilt. That reminded me it was my duty to take care of myself because being a good mom was all I wanted to be.

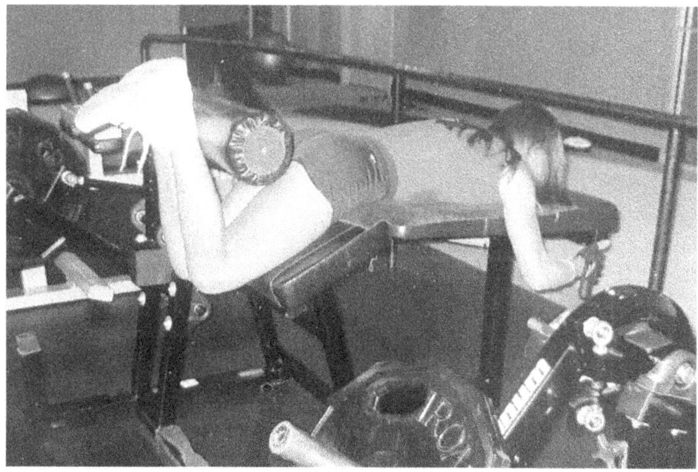

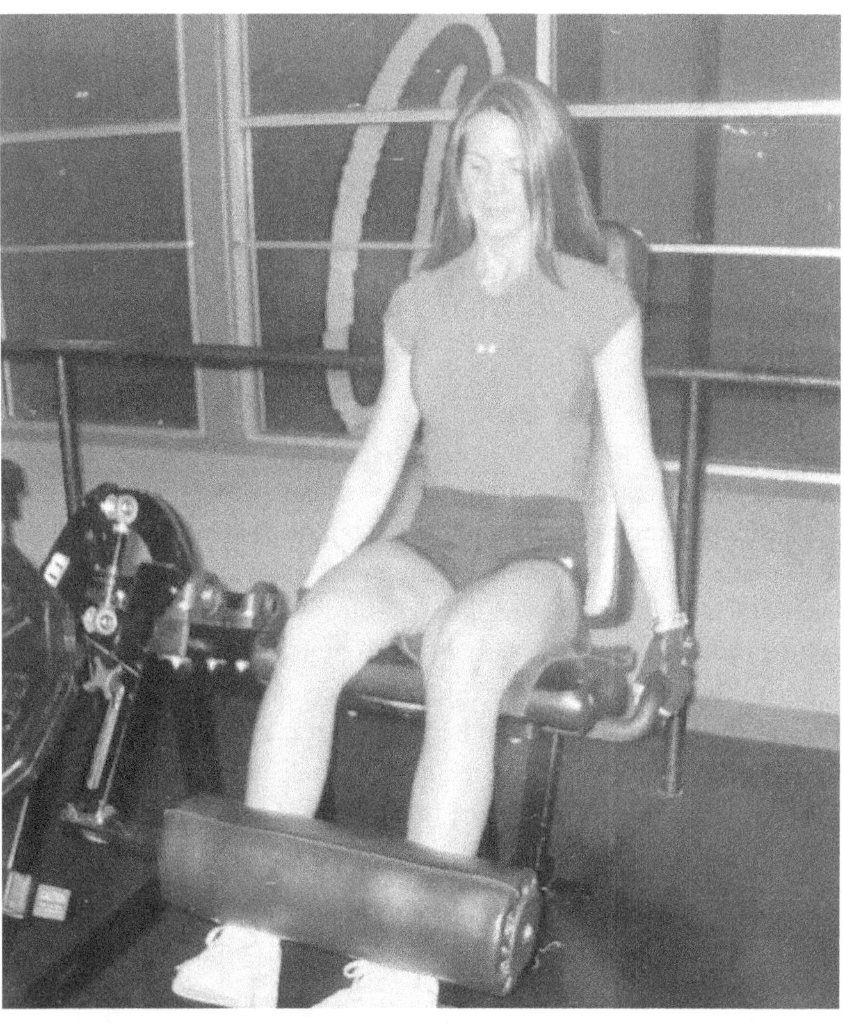

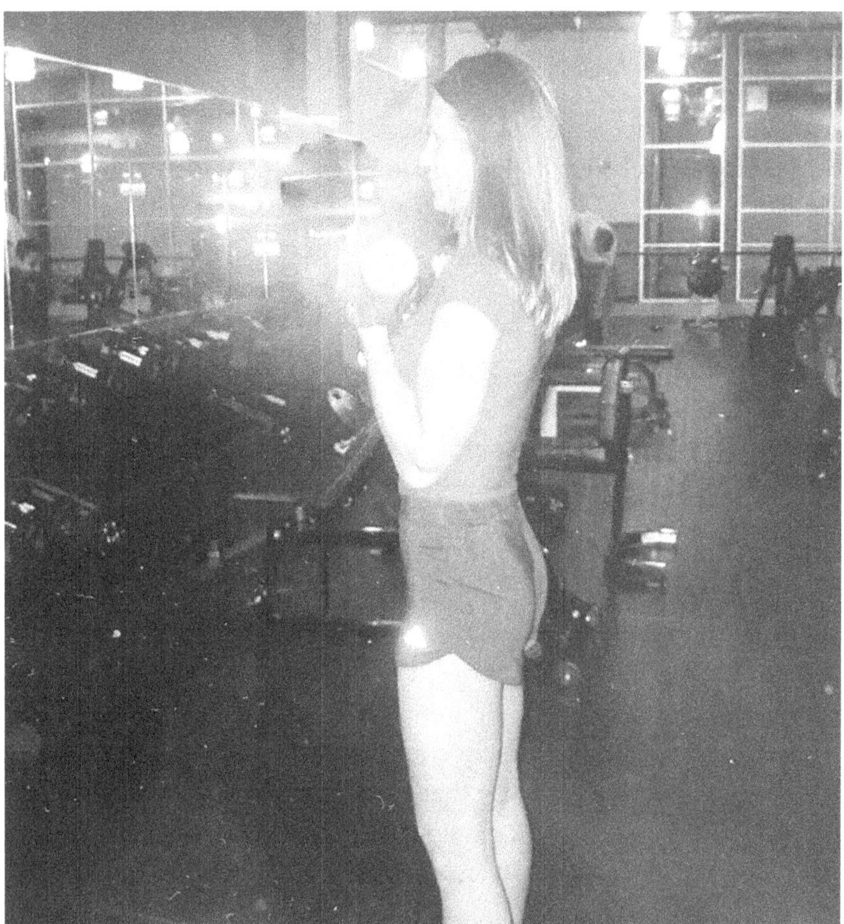

This is about one year into my workout program. I lost body fat, but had not gained a whole lot of muscle yet. I was still curling 8lb dumbbells. I started my personal training career shortly after these were taken. I came along way at this point, but it was just the beginning for me.

For better or worse, that phrase justified my sneaking around to go to the gym because all I was really doing was taking the path of least resistance to accomplish a goal. I was not going to get my husband's support. And I was at the point where his support truly was no longer important to me. That reflects who and what he was during that time. It was not a reflection on me and the woman I was becoming. He was insecure at that time, and, as it turned out, rightfully so. Quite frankly, I did not want the argument.

I continued doing what I wanted, and it made Joey crazy. I was still babysitting for kids during the day, and I was still doing gift backets at night in between homework and classes, but my workouts continued, and I believe Joey could not take any more of my "independence." That was right about the time I decided to have my boobs done as a treat to myself. I thought after ALL the money he blew on his bad choices; I could spend money on this. And it was the best money I ever spent. Not only did he go into a high-speed wobble at this time, but my friends and family went with him. Most of them, not all of them, but most of them thought I was being extremely irrational.

By this point, there was not one person who did not suspect me of having an affair. All the signs pointed in that direction, but this was also about the time that I realized that once people make up their minds about something, there's no sense in trying to change it. I realized that the ones who were judging me were the ones I should care less about, not more. In fact, most of them could have been categorized as being hypocritical on the subject, so that made me care even less what they thought. I stopped answering questions about it and I stopped engaging with people who I felt were cornering me. I was non-compliant, arrogant, confident, and could care less who judged me. I had spent too many years of my life trying to get shitty people to like me, treat me well, and understand me. And I was done.

I will admit that I was being a huge bitch to Joey. Not because I went out one day to get my boobs done, but because my attitude toward him finally caught up to all the negative emotions I had had for so many years. He was no longer getting a reaction out of me with his shitty comments, and he really had no idea how to handle me not caring when he stayed out all night. He eventually moved out of our home and moved in with one of my stepbrothers. My family members and some friends thought I lost my mind letting him go. But I felt a huge weight finally lifted off my shoulders—a weight I had been carrying alone for years. Relief is the only way to explain what I felt then. I felt like I now had a fighting chance to make a difference in my life and for my kids' lives.

I started asking myself this simple question when people judged me, "Will I ever have to report to them?" If the answer was, "No" (and it usually was), then I didn't give a shit what they thought of me. It was magical. It was empowering. And it was long overdue.

My mother, God bless her, was put in the middle of this. Since Joey was crying on my stepbrother's shoulders and they were telling my stepdad everything, my mom was left to hear about it at the dinner table and at family functions that I long since stopped attending. I felt badly for her, but I simply could not protect anyone else for any longer. I needed to take care of me and my girls. That's it.

The irony wasn't lost on me though that he was crying on the shoulders of some of the least sensitive men in the greater Chicago area. Some of them were involved with his bad behavior and bad decisions and could be rightfully accused of encouraging it. Using my family as a support group was completely out of line.

Right around this time, my mom was having regular talks with me after the Sunday family get-togethers. She would remind me what this might do to the kids, what it might do to me financially, and on and on. It was all the normal things someone who loves you and cares about your well-being would say. She was afraid for me, and rightfully so. But I remember distinctly telling her once I could no longer take it, "Mom, you are either WITH ME or you are AGAINST me."

She paused, looked at me in my eyes, and said, "You are right. You are my daughter. No matter if you are doing right, wrong, or otherwise, you are my daughter and I back you 100%."

That was the last time she tried to change my position and I loved her even more for it. I let her in on my five-year plan. She had had no idea how unhappy I was for so long. She lived with similar circumstances with her husband and so after so many years, this behavior just seemed normal from her perspective. But I refused to accept this approach as "my normal." It was not normal to me—it was wrong. I was better than that and I was going to be damned if I was not going to start being treated with some fucking respect. There was only one person in charge of how I was going to be treated. I could beg, plead, cry, throw things … it didn't matter. I learned that when someone does not want to change, they are not going to change, so I had to make some changes myself.

Chapter 19

ENDINGS AND NEW BEGINNINGS

A couple of months after Joey moved out of the house, I filed for divorce. I had set aside money from the last time we refinanced for the attorney's retainer—I knew, deep down, it would come to this. It was part of the five-year plan, and the only way I would ever have access to thousands of dollars to pay an attorney all at one time. Then I used any money from my business to pay our everyday expenses and for the new car I bought. There was never extra money on hand at that time.

The day I received my divorce papers in the mail from my attorney was probably one of the darkest days of my life. Fortunately, the kids were with Joey the entire day because I stayed in bed crying all day long. You would think after the way he treated me I would be jumping for joy. Instead, I felt like such a failure. I felt sorry for myself, wondering why could he not change those things that were dragging our family down so badly? Why could he not stop drinking for his wife and his daughters? Why could he not stop gambling away our future? Endings … and new beginnings … are fraught with emotion, not logic, though. We simply have to go through it to get to the other side.

One thing was clear to me. He just didn't love me like I loved him, at least not enough to give some things up for our future. That's a slap in the face, even when there are red flags along the way. But suddenly, it was all very clear. As disappointed as I was, the decisions he had made were hurtful, and it was real, and it was the truth.

The next morning, I was headed to Florida to stay with my mom and stepfather for a week at their winter home. I had the kids with me, and my divorce papers. Joey called me just before we boarded our flight and asked if we could please make another go at it. He said he finally realized what he needed to do to change. He realized what I had been saying all these years. I couldn't believe my ears. Could I really believe him this time? Did he mean it? When I started to sway to *maybe* and then to *maybe* and then to *yes*, I found myself both relieved and excited.

I told him how I could not get myself out of bed because I was so depressed and second guessing this life-changing decision. I still loved him so much and I thought he was actually going to start incorporating the things our marriage counselor had gone over with us, such as putting me and the kids first. It took very little for him to convince me he was a changed man because he was saying everything I really wanted to hear.

He had me in the palm of his hand. And he knew it. He said he could not wait until we got back from Florida so we could talk about things. I really believed we could hold it together. I thought he was finally taking me seriously and he was going to see that it was time to grow up. But before the end of the call, I realized how mistaken I was.

As I was imagining our happily ever after once again, Joey said, "Oh yeah, by the way, the night you get back from Florida, I am supposed to have the kids, but I have plans that night. One of my friends is playing in a band at the House of Blues and I really want to go."

Not sure I heard him right and giving him a chance to make the situation right, I replied, "But you won't have seen the kids for an entire week, and they will want to see you."

"I know, but my friend is playing, and I want to see him."

"So, it doesn't matter that your kids want to see you, because you want to see your friends instead? The same friends you see all the time."

"Well, yes, but he's playing at the House of Blues. This is a pretty big deal for him!"

"I need to go," I said, hanging up the phone.

I was absolutely shocked. I am not sure why, but I was. He had me thinking for a few short moments that he was going to start putting our family first—not his friends, but our family. He couldn't even get through one single phone conversation before his true colors and intentions showed. This was a crucial time for us, and he just couldn't find it in his heart to do it. It was at that moment that I knew I had to make the hardest decision of my life. I didn't want to make this decision, but he was leaving me with no choice. I tried everything I could to fix us, but we were too far broken. I had to take the emotion out of it and when I did, I realized I just had to make a business decision for my family.

The shock began to morph into acceptance by the time we boarded the plane. But acceptance or not, I was sick the whole way there. I didn't know if I was relieved that I was getting out of the limbo I had been in for so long, as hard as it was going to be, or if I was sad that it was so obvious that he was not capable of changing. When my mom picked us up from the airport, she looked at me and asked, "What's the matter? You look like you just saw a ghost."

She could see it on my face. She didn't know what was wrong, but she knew something was off. I told her what happened on the phone right before we boarded. She couldn't hide her disappointment and then anger. She was actually yelling, while she was driving, "What is wrong with him!? He had you in the palm of his hand! I cannot believe he could do something so stupid! He is losing you and doesn't even seem to care! I don't understand!"

I know exactly what she was feeling and thinking because I had been thinking and feeling this for years! I finally felt like someone was understanding me, which in its own way, was comforting. No matter what we go through, and no matter how strong we are, the comfort and support provided by a loved one in a time of need is invaluable.

Two of my stepbrothers were also in Florida at the time and when they heard what had happened, they continued to try to talk me into staying with him. One of them was trying to justify Joey as always, "You know how he is! Not a mean bone in his body, he's just being Joey!" Suddenly, I saw the light and it was clear. I was almost relieved. Depressed, but relieved. Yes, I did know how he was and that was not good enough for me. Period.

The rest of the trip felt like I was just going through the motions with my daughters and family. My mind and my heart just weren't in it. I was thinking about how the girls were going to take the news. I can't even remember when or where I was, or how I told them what was about to happen. I feel as if I blacked out or was in a dream (or nightmare) during this part of my life. It was too painful to anticipate how my little girls would react. I returned home the following weekend. My husband went out with his friends instead of taking our girls for the weekend, and I signed the papers and returned them to my lawyer.

For the next several months, when Joey would have the kids on the weekends, I would periodically go out with friends. I was at an event with old high school friends who I had not seen in years, and I had asked Nate if he wanted to come along. He agreed, and we were having a nice time. By chance, one of Joey's friends was also at the event. I said hello to him and was met with a look of disgust. Oh well, I wasn't going to waste a second thinking about it.

Later that night, someone came up behind me and grabbed a fist full of hair from my scalp. Then, he whispered in my ear, "We need to talk."

I turned around and saw it was this friend. I asked him in a *"who the hell do you think you are,"* tone, "About what?" He gave me another dirty look and walked away. Once again, I wasn't going to waste my energy on this childish crap.

Nate and I left shortly thereafter. Once we got in the car, I told him what had happened. He was calm but angry. I didn't tell him on the spot because I knew exactly how he would have handled it and I didn't want to make a scene. I did, however, call Joey first thing in the morning to tell him that his friend better hope he doesn't run into Nate again. Joey swore he knew nothing about it and apologized for it happening. Later, he confirmed that his friend was pretty proud of acting this way, but Joey reminded him how that could have ended had I not been a better person. I had to drop it because this friend of Joey's worked at the golf course that Joey managed. I knew he would be around my girls, and I did not want him mistreating them.

For Joey's family functions, I would always drop the girls off, so they could still have a relationship with his side of the family (even though he wouldn't attend because of work or whatever). On a number of occasions, I was snubbed by his family, as I walked my kids into the event to make sure they got off ok. I would say hello and ask certain people how they were, trying to make small talk, and I would be ignored or made to feel out of place. Meanwhile, my family was not only friendly with Joey, but a couple of them invited him to move in with them, making ME feel like the outsider … in my own family. I guess nothing new there, though.

While I was going through the divorce, I was being shit talked and mistreated by his family and friends, I had to watch my family take him under their wings, I was desperately trying to finish up my classes, I was running the basket business, and I was raising three little girls. I remember once my mother asking me how the hell I was keeping everything straight. And to be honest, I was not sure, but I think that was about the time that I realized that the more I hated things in my world, the busier I made myself. I would get laser focused on not pertaining to the things that hurt me the most. I guess it's my defense mechanism—my coping mechanism. And during that time, I hated him most. I could have never anticipated the good relationship he and I would develop by 2018.

One of the ways I dealt with the stress threatening me and my health was by hitting the gym. Hard. I started taking my training very seriously. I committed to an entirely new healthy lifestyle. I cut out bread and pasta (making my Italian family question my sanity even more), fruit after 5:00 p.m., and alcohol completely (another deal breaker with my family). My body was responding well to the program, and I started feeling healthier and more clear-headed, than I ever had in my life.

I started spending more time with Nate outside the club. He helped me with things around the house—fixed my broken lawn mower, helped me go through my expenses to see where I could cut things, etc. One day, he ran to a pharmacy to pick up medication when all three of my girls were sick with sore throats and fevers. He even snuck in three tubs of Ben and Jerry's ice cream for them! He was as supportive as always and continued to help me build my confidence and support my wants and needs. He helped me come to terms with the fact that just because people are family does not mean they are good people. I adopted the idea from him that, "I don't know," is a perfectly good answer. And the word, "No," does not need an explanation. These are all things that made me believe in myself … and in him.

One night, while he was repairing my washing machine, my 9-year-old, asked him, "Do you like my mommy?" I heard it through the door from the next room. My jaw dropped and my eyes widened. I thought, "Oh my God…what is she doing?"

He answered, "Yes, I like your mommy."

She continued, "Maybe you can take her out on a date?"

It was one of the cutest things she ever did. And God Bless her for watching over her mommy! I was nervous at that because I had started liking him but held back because I wasn't sure it was for all the right reasons. He seemed to rescue me from a really bad situation, but I wanted to like him for him, not for being a white knight in some fucked up fairy tale. As he was leaving, he gathered all the girls in front of him, along with me, and asked them if it would be okay to take me out on a date. My 6-year-old answered yes reluctantly, but in the end, they all gave their blessing, and we made dinner plans for that weekend.

It felt like my first real adult date … and it was. This date was like a fantasy come true—kind of like a Cinderella movie. He showed up with a bag of clothes and a pair of boots from expensive stores where I would never dream of shopping. He came into my house and said, "You look great, and I am sure you took a lot of time picking out your outfit, but I thought you might want to wear something new."

He handed over the bags. In them was a hot pink Italian leather crop jacket, with black leather pants, leather boots with a very short heel, and two leather purses, pink and black, so I could pick which one I thought went better with the outfit. I was shocked and amazed. What a thoughtful man—a man who took care of me and wanted me to feel good about myself. I didn't even know a man like that existed.

What I loved even more than how he treated me though was how good he was to my kids. Over the next several months, he became the father figure they needed. He was the one who read them books before bed. He was the one who helped them with their homework. They saw him respecting me and treating me like a lady. He opened our car doors, all of us. He pulled out my chair at breakfast, lunch, and dinner. He walked street side. He had the class and manors I had never seen before … except, of course, from my dad.

He made me feel secure for the first time I remembered since my dad, when I was a little girl. It was such a relief. It was like I was being rescued.

Chapter 20

A NEW CAREER

I finally graduated from DePaul University In 2003. *I owe it all to my dad* might be too strong a statement to attribute this huge milestone to, but if it weren't for him being so adamant, I am not sure I would have had the drive to do it in some of the most stressful times of my life. I had to prove to him that I could do it, but more importantly, I had to show my kids what determination and persistence look like. I had to walk in graduation. I had to. I had to wait for them to call my name, shake their hands, take my degree, kiss it, and hold it up to the heavens in thanks. My mom and kids were there, and that made me so proud. None of my sisters had graduated from college, so I knew my mom was elated.

Next in my plan was looking for a full-time job. I went to a recruiter for help and made the decision to dissolve the basket business. Looking back, I should have tried to sell it. It had real value to it, but there was just too much going on at the time to even consider that. I wouldn't have even known where to start. The internet was around, but I was not good at knowing the power of it. So, after several years of building, what I considered, a successful small business, All Occasion Baskets closed its doors. And that's okay. Sometimes, we need to walk away from things that no longer serve us or are an integral part of another time in our lives. That's what this was. I needed closure in every aspect from that time in my life.

I realized after I had been on an interview or two in corporate America that I really did not fit in. The interviews that I went on made me feel like I had a third eye, just walking through the office space to get to the interview with the person in charge. I dressed professionally for the interviews, and I was in really good shape physically. I wasn't sure if maybe the women in the office didn't like how I looked. Or maybe they were worried because I had kids at home? One of the interviewers actually expressed that if one of my kids was sick at home, she wasn't sure that I would handle it properly. And she was a mother! It was like they would use any excuse to hide how they really felt about me.

One day, one of the women in a small cubicle got the attention of another one and they both stared at me as I was walking out. I saw them, and they made me feel very uncomfortable. I'd like to give them the benefit of the doubt, but I had also learned by then to trust my instincts. I knew it was not going to be a good fit. I didn't go back.

After some consideration about what to do next, I asked Nate for some advice. I had been training with him for a year and trusted his judgment. I asked him if he thought I should go for my certification and become a Certified Personal Trainer. He excitedly answered yes, telling me that the knowledge I had gained from him came directly from the United States government, and that there is no better resource. He thought I would be better prepared than other trainers for that reason alone.

So, I did it. I took my training knowledge to the next level and decided to make it a career. After I finished my college degree in business and nutrition, I took my first certification in personal training. Once my certification was complete, it was time to start asking for interviews. I went to the club in Bloomingdale where I worked out most often and the manager there interviewed me. I thought it was a slam dunk! A month later, I still had not heard anything from him. Even with two follow up calls, he said he had not yet made a decision.

One day, I decided to go workout at a different club from the same chain. I stood out because of how fit I was and happened to start talking with the personal training director there. She asked me if I would come back the next day for an interview. I did, and she hired me on the spot. It was not the club of my choice because it was further from my house, but I was thrilled.

The very next morning, I received a phone call from the manager at the Bloomingdale location. He, "heard the news," and was *not* happy I took the position at the other location. I asked him to explain his position, as I had waited over a month for an answer from him. He had nothing to say. He was clearly pissed, and rude actually, but offered me to come there instead. I declined and started at the other location the following week. Once again, I trusted my instincts, as we all need to do more often. I saw his character by the way he strung me along, while making me squirm and practically beg for a job. There was no way working for him would be any better.

Over the next six years, that manager from Bloomingdale came into our location weekly. And he would take every chance he got to shoot me a dirty look. The first couple of times, I tried to say hello, assuming he would be professional, but he snubbed me. He had no idea that it would take a lot more than a snub to rattle me. And every quarter, when the numbers came out and my PT Director was exceeding goals based on my training sales, she couldn't have been happier with her decision, and neither could I. She was going on company trips two times a year and her salary doubled within six months of me starting.

I cannot take all the credit for the success of that club though. A few months after I started at that location, Nate retired from the government job and was approached by the PT director to take a position as a personal trainer. She ran it past me first, as by now he and I were dating, and she did not want me to be uncomfortable if we worked together.

I was reluctant because I had started to suspect that he was a bit controlling. It seemed like he wanted to spend every spare minute I had with him, which was the exact opposite of what I was used to with Joey. If I had something else to do that didn't include him, he seemed to get irritable. I was beginning to worry that I was getting into another bad relationship, but he convinced me that it was me who wasn't used to compromise and that was the reason for the issues we were having.

I believed him and thought a little compromise on my part was okay. As far as the job, I knew the more I rode his coat tails and listened and learned from him, the better I would be, so I figured the hands-on training would be great for my career. This was a very rare opportunity that I had to continue to learn from one of the best in terms of training. Still, I weighed the pros and cons of being together a little too much, but thought the good would outweigh the bad, so I agreed to have him come to the same location as a trainer.

We started working together and were killing it. We worked well as a team because he had a background that was so unique and impressive, and I was the perfect prototype example of what our program could do in such little time. Our schedules were booking up faster than we could take on new clients. We both had a three-month waitlist to get on our schedules. Within one month of him starting, he was the #1 trainer nationwide, out of 4,500 trainers, and I was #2 (#1 female.) We held this position for YEARS—no one could come close. I was making the top trainer list month after month and all the big wigs across the country from this club chain knew my name. I won incentives and trips based on my sales. It was crazy, like being a celebrity in my own little community.

My girls were starting to get used to my new schedule. They handled it well, considering I went from a stay-at-home mom to fifteen-hour days in less than two years. It was gradual, but it was real. I would get home to pick them up from school, get them home to do homework, feed them dinner, then get back to work for the evening while I had other friends' moms, or my sister drive them to gymnastics.

During the divorce, I got to keep the house, which was important to me, so the kids wouldn't feel so much change at once, but I had to absorb the

$80,000 in credit card debt from the lifestyle Joey led as a trade-off for that decision. Working off this debt meant long hours, plain and simple. Plus, I got so much out of my work. I felt fulfilled and happy to be helping others achieve their goals. At one point, my girls mentioned they didn't like it. I wanted them to know that I would be there for them, but I also took on this financial responsibility that meant I had no choice. So, I tried to put it into perspective for them. I told them if we could cut back on a few things here and there, I could probably cut my hours a bit. But my main responsibility was being able to provide for them in every way possible, including staying in our home, and that meant I had to work hard.

Nonetheless, the schedule eventually began to wear on me. Yes, I was getting my debt paid down, but my schedule was building so fast that it was becoming overwhelming. My kids were still little, eleven and nine, but life was passing me by. Time with my mom was also extremely limited, and I hated that. We used to talk every day when I was a stay-at-home mom. I barely had time to talk to her every few days now.

Joey went on to immediately move in with his new girlfriend, who quickly turned into his fiancé within a year. That devastated me more than I thought it would. He called me at work one day to tell me he got engaged, and I broke down in tears. He felt so badly, not knowing I would take the news as I did. I just couldn't help but think that maybe he was going to change and someone else would get the man that I waited for all those years. But most importantly, that conversation allowed me to let go.

Chapter 21

FRIEND OR FOE?

We weren't even with the company six months before we were invited to speak every other month at the Personal Trainer's New Recruits Boot Camp Week. This event was a one-week boot camp and sales technique class to teach the trainers how to effectively sell training. The manager from the Bloomingdale location and his top trainer spoke at this event for years, but now the district manager for all of Chicagoland asked us to speak too. He wanted us to talk about how we were able to sell so much personal training continuously month after month after month.

We let the Bloomingdale manager and his top trainer go first. Then we went. Our approach was so different, our energy on another level—and the whole room could feel it. The Bloomingdale manager and his trainer ultimately came across as used car salesmen, while we came in with a program that sold itself because it was based on the math and biology of the human body. The basis of our speech was that most people are simply doing it wrong because they don't know any better. They don't understand how the body works. We would use my experience as a prime example. And we ended with how we did our jobs to give clients the answers they needed. That was what separated us from the rest.

We would, "Wow," these new recruits every time we spoke. Trainers would ask if they could come from other clubs just to shadow us to try to learn our program. We were quite a force—and quite a team. But again, making it very difficult to break away. We came in as two people who knew we could make a difference in people's lives. We made it clear that if you could take care of people and make a change in their lives, you would be successful personal trainers.

I wish I could say that it was the working together, living together, and raising my daughters together that caused the huge strain on our relationship, but looking back, that is not what it was at all. He was a unique person, who claimed to see rare things while working for the government. He seemed to be suffering from something that I could not understand. But I did understand the results of it—I noticed him becoming very controlling and demanding of my time. If I would try to get time away, even to go see my mom or my girls without him, once I arrived home, he would act sad and/or mad and sometimes give me the silent treatment. At times, his needy behavior was unbearable. I remember wondering why there can't just be a happy medium—my ex-husband never wanted to be with me, and my new boyfriend wouldn't give me a minute to myself.

We were at the club together for about two years when I knew, without a doubt, that I had to get out of this relationship. But these things are hard to do, especially when you work with your partner every day. Several more years ticked on, where I felt like I was on a rollercoaster with him. I knew all along that the bad was bad, and completely unacceptable. That didn't make it any easier to break away, though. Every time he made a mistake, he would do something GRAND like remodel a room in my house, or buy me a Corvette, or something. You know, things I could not do for myself. The bigger the offense, the bigger the gift. I believe there is a name for this…love bombing. But then those mistakes became much more than mistakes.

I was always wondering where the man I fell in love with went. When was he coming back? He would show signs of being back, then he'd do something that I would consider, *questionable* again. This cycle went on for years. But, by that point, I couldn't see a way out.

Many clients, trainers, and co-workers witnessed the behavior and the dynamics of our relationship that I endured during this time. If he was mad at me about something, and I mean anything, he wasn't one to wait to get home to discuss it. He would approach me, even with clients, every chance he had. It got to a point where any time he would walk toward me while I was with a client, they knew it was going to be a *talking to* for me. He would start with, "Can I talk to you for a minute?" in a condescending tone. Even if I would tell him, "It will have to wait until we get home," he would not hesitate to say what was on his mind right then and there. It felt like he got a rise out of putting on a show for them. I would do my best to brush it off, but there were times that he would push me to my limit, and I would completely lose it. A scene was caused in the gym at least once a week. It was so embarrassing. And then he would follow up every argument with a very nice gift—even my clients noticed the pattern.

I threatened to break up with him more times than I can count. And at times, I did. But he reminded me that he was the reason I had any clients and that because he was technically higher up than me in the club, they would keep him, and I would be out. I believed him. He would tell me things like, "Good luck building your schedule all over again, hahaha!" Honestly, this is the only reason I stayed. I knew how hard I had to work to build what I had, and I didn't believe I could do it again, at the same time I would be raising my daughters on my own. I fell into the trap of not believing I was strong enough to leave. Again. How did I let this happen? Again.

It blows my mind that I was convinced of this because before he came along, I had a ton of stress and horrible situations to deal with, and I was able to make it on my own. Why the hell couldn't I do it now? Well, of course, I could, but the confidence that was once built up was now once again destroyed by someone I loved. And when we're in that state, our minds can be manipulated.

As our popularity grew, this chain wanted more of the cut, and before long, we realized it was time to take our show on the road. We leased space at a smaller gym in the area, and out of ninety clients between us, eighty-nine of them followed. And it was nothing personal with the one who didn't—it was a location issue with her work schedule.

We were working as a team, and in true Linda fashion, I buried myself in work to keep my mind busy. In this way, I didn't have time to think about my personal life. I was so mad at myself though, knowing that this was the perfect point for me to escape this relationship. But because I was so confused as to how to transition my clients to this new club, I stayed and watched and learned from him. This was like nothing I ever had to coordinate before, and unless you have had to do it, you may not understand how it can be like herding cats.

Business at this new club was doing great. They were thrilled that they were getting a very nice percentage of our monthly sales, but I felt even more trapped, as we were now truly growing a business together. This new club asked us to oversee their training program in the entire Chicago area. We took on seven clubs within the first year, training trainers to get them up to a reasonable standard with our program and place them at their own clubs. We had two trainers at each club, but this club chain also wanted more of the cut, like the last, and started to make business decisions that were uncomfortable to me. We needed to break away. After a two-year run there, we decided to bring all our trainers under one roof and open our own location in Elk Grove Village, Illinois.

The building of this club, both the actual buildout and then building a membership base, was very time consuming and stressful. But we were also having some fun! We really became a team with the trainers who were working for us. We hired these trainers based on character, not based on what they knew, so they were good people who had great senses of humor. We would tell them to forget everything they knew before, as we didn't want to have to try to go against bad habits or stupid things that they read on the internet while they were retraining in our program.

My daughters started working for us, and for a time, I couldn't have been happier! They had a difficult time with it at first because they had some serious responsibilities now, with it being their first job. We held them to a very high standard. But I was so happy that I could see their faces every day they were there. It helped them build confidence and a good work ethic.

The behavior that Nate displayed in front of clients at our original club continued at our club though. And the unfortunate part of my daughters being there was that they were now witnessing it all firsthand. I tried to hide it the best I could, like I did at home, but they knew. They were usually at the front desk or cleaning while he was instigating me by my clients, so I counted on them not seeing a lot of it. It was still unbearable for me at times, and the roller coaster ride continued. Bad behavior followed up with amazing gifts. Never an apology, just gifts.

Three years after we built our first club, our second club opened. And more than anything, it was such a huge relief for me, as I was able to be away from him and escape that trapped feeling being with him all day, every day. Even my twin daughters were scheduled at the Des Plaines location. They were eighteen at the time and certified personal trainers, as well. They started to build up their own clientele there.

Yet, at times, it did not matter that I was not at the same club as him. He called constantly to yell at me for any reason he could find every chance he could get. The stress of opening the new location seemed to have thrown him over the edge. I felt like he became more and more unruly and more easily irritated. Thankfully, only the verbal incidents increased. The vulgar name calling was unbearable at times. To me, he was the one adding to all the stress, just by the way he acted.

Remember the five-year-plan I had with my ex-husband? I wish I could say I had the same plan at that time, but I didn't. I searched for a way to get out of this, what could be considered, toxic relationship but had no idea how. The club was in his name and the equipment was in mine. I would need him to agree to sell to me, or for me to rent another location and just move my equipment out, but I would need accountants and attorneys on this, and it all seemed so overwhelming to me. I am not sure how I could have made it all work. It was too risky to go and rent another location alone. And I knew he would not go along with any of this, especially if it meant me leaving him, so it would be costly.

I was surprised that once again, I was getting hung up on attempting to control someone else's behavior. Hadn't I learned that it is impossible to do that already? And, of course, the confusion set in because as bad as it could be, my experience was that the highs were so very high that people on the outside were completely envious.

Special days and holidays were ruined because of his behavior. My youngest daughter, suffered the most. She was a back-talker, and he tried to teach her a lesson every step of the way, making our home life very difficult. The twins were very compliant and usually did whatever it took not to set him off. Although they experienced the rollercoaster effect of living with him, fortunately they were at school, gymnastics, their dad's and at work most of their lives.

They did not witness the name calling, but they did witness the silent treatment he gave me. The silent treatment was when he was mad at me, and I wouldn't give in to the ridiculousness. It also showed up if I called him out on something that he did, which I guess he hated. I dealt with the silent treatment my entire childhood from my stepfather, so I could deal with it now as an adult. Plus, I had the satisfaction of knowing it was harder for him than it was me.

To me, he always looked like he was so angry, like he was going to blow at any minute. I think it was a scare tactic, but we would all just roll our eyes at him—after all, what else can you do at times? I looked at that silent treatment like a break from him, but my kids knew it was wrong and it often made them feel very uncomfortable, as if they did something wrong. So, he would try to be extra nice to them, probably so they would think I was the problem. But they knew—my girls are smart.

I took a step back and looked at my situation and saw the way this all might have been affecting my daughters. I couldn't help but think about my mom and the similar situation she faced while married to my step-father. I now had a much better understanding of her decision to stay. It was not so much a decision, as much as it was survival. She felt stuck. He made her life great at times, too. I swore I would never let my kids go through the same treatment, but I have guilt, every day that I might have failed in that respect.

Chapter 22

LINDA STEELE, THE BRAND

At the same time the Des Plaines location was going up, the "Linda Steele" brand was born. Nate realized that there was no way we could keep up in this highly competitive industry without embracing social media. And even though we were years behind on this trend, we made a go at it.

Nate knew we were unique with our training and his background, and we had a huge local following, but he knew he could grow that bigger and better with social media. Since I was "the draw," in so many ways, he used me, my name, and my personality to build a major social media presence, inextricably tying me to him even further. I was reluctant to get onboard, however, because as much as I loved dressing up and had a unique flair about me, I wasn't sure I could be "all that" to the public. My friends and family knew me to be fun, sweet, and confident, but being an influencer meant being "in your face," and that wasn't really me.

Anyone familiar with social media influencers knows that a huge part of a presence is taking selfies. I think I took my first selfie in 2017, about two years after we started being active, then my second one, probably a year or so after. I absolutely hated them and could not understand how anyone could be so vain. It wasn't until about 2020 that I started taking them on a regular basis. I also had a hard time sharing my day-to-day activities. I wondered who the hell would care what I was doing. But, as it turns out, a lot of people cared! And if I wanted to make this worth my while, I'd better share all about it.

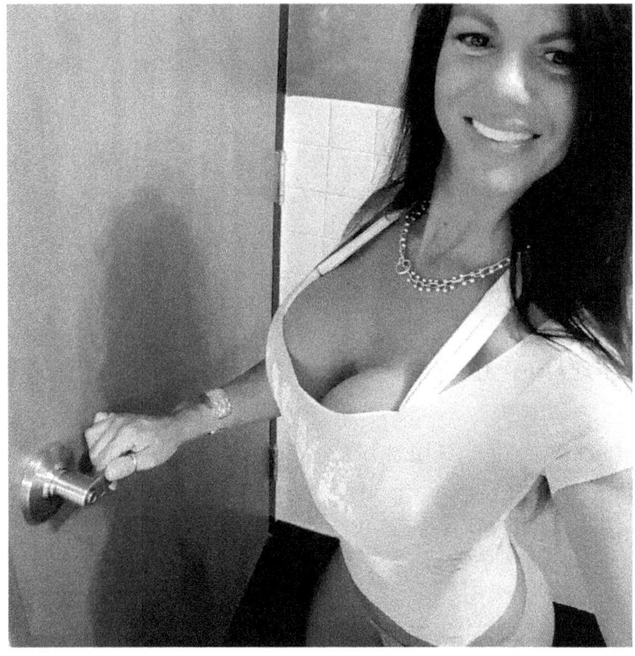

This was my very first selfie. It took a number of takes because I was trying to figure out how to hold the camera and take the picture with your same hand!

My girls were behind me, helping to build my following and my social media likes and comments. It took a while for them to get used to the idea of me strutting around in bikinis for men all over the world to watch. They were similar to kids who grew up before the 90s, when kids didn't get to share their opinions, but more than that, they were extremely respectful and trusted the decisions that I made. Because it was out of character for me to do those things, I did talk to them about it and remind them that a beautiful body is what I worked for, and this happened to be a business decision. They eventually looked it as business and were able to separate it from daughters seeing their mom in these types of photos on social media. They got it.

There was one occasion, however, when I drove up to pick them up from school and they were wrestling on the ground with a boy claiming to be defending me. "You should have heard what he said about you!" I had to remind them that it was a business. They eventually matured, and so did the boys, and it all settled in. My daughters are still friends with the same boys from elementary school and high school, and they have shown nothing but the utmost respect for me to this day.

I went along with all the attention, and I started being contacted by photographers as soon as they got word. Nate put me on the Model Mayhem website to start. Modeling had been something that I always wanted to do once I got into shape. I wasn't sure how long I could maintain it, to be honest, and I wanted a record of looking the way I did. I put so much effort into it and saw a transformation that I never thought I could attain.

One photoshoot turned into another, and before I knew it, I was being approached by promoters in Los Angeles, celebrity photographers, musicians, and people in the sports and entertainment industry who did photography as a second job or hobby. I was being contacted internationally from radio stations and magazines to co-host and be part of their shows. I couldn't even take advantage of all the opportunities because I had two businesses to run at home and several clients to work with six to seven days a week. My schedule was still starting every day at 5:00 a.m. and going until about 10:00 p.m.

Eventually, I did start traveling and making it to events to which I was invited. At one point, I had photo shoots scheduled once a month everywhere from Nashville to Miami to Tampa to Vegas and California. While I still had to turn down shoots due to my "real job," the ones I did make it to gave me a ton of content to start my website. That was the idea, after all. To make money. Getting paid for the photoshoots was great, but it was not going to allow me to quit my day job, by any means. So, how does a social media influencer monetize all of his or her followers? By directing the followers to something they are willing to pay for! We had to find something that people would find valuable.

My website offered nutrition plans, workout plans, posters from some of the photo shoots, as well as a paid subscription section that provided access to exclusive photos, they would not find on my social media platforms. A lot of these photos were from my bikini shoots from companies who sponsored me, as well. That being said, a whole lot of skin was being shown on my website, and I was getting a really nice, supportive following.

The more that social media followers responded to the photos showing more skin, the more of those types of photos Nate posted. When he posted the brilliant articles I wrote about carbohydrates for instance, I would get about 100 likes. When he posted a bikini photo, I would get 1,000 likes. I became very uncomfortable with these bikini photos being posted because it just came on so fast. I was about ten years removed from severe body dysmorphia, where I spent a lot of time worrying about flaws in my appearance, and it was still a lot to process. Being proud of the way I looked was one thing but being under the microscope while wearing a microscopic swimsuit is another!

But this was a fast left turn from what we had discussed about the brand being born. We had talked about going down the road of a personal trainer and nutrition expert by showing off the product of a healthy lifestyle, not a bikini model, so I was *not* prepared for the direction this was going. I didn't demand to stay on track because he and I both had a business mindset, and I could see why he was doing it. And I am glad I made these decision—fitness trainers and nutrition experts are a dime a dozen. I wanted to be more.

I rarely went on my social media because I was too busy, so there were plenty of days in a row I wouldn't even see the photos or the comments, but a client would mention them to me. That was a bit awkward, but to make Nate not look so much like he was pushing me in this direction, I found myself defending his choice of photos posted. As I mentioned, I understood what he was doing. I understood he was following the lead of the viewers and what they wanted to see, so my pages would build. This is a fine line when building a social media following. It is a hard needle to thread. It's important to give followers what they want, but to do so without losing yourself, your voice, and your original goal can be a supreme challenge.

About a year or so into my brand, I was approached by an online fitness platform named Fit.Live. It was owned by AJ Joshi, one of the UK's most influential entrepreneurs. And he invited me to be on his show, which went out to about nine different social media platforms. I did the workout show three times per week, and I taught my program to viewers all over the world.

I would have anywhere from 10,000 to 50,000 viewers on every show. It was eye-opening and so fun for me to be able to interact with so many people at once. This also broadened my exposure in the international market, leading me to meet Stewart St. Claire and becoming part of UK Health Radio and writing health and fitness articles for UK Health Triangle.

Then, about a year or so into Fit.Live, I was approached by Brian Sebastian, a promoter in LA, and founder of Movie Reviews and More, which just made "Top 50 Podcasts" in Forbes. That landed me a co-host position on I Heart Radio, Women on TV, LA Talk Radio, and 4KTV, just to name a few. I was working side by side with actors, popular models, and famous inventors. This expanded my exposure even more. Professionally, things were looking up.

I made some great friends on this journey. These men worked closely by my side and pushed to get my brand out there to help build my following. While dealing with me, they also dealt with Nate, and watched my personal struggles with him. They were there at the photoshoots and saw the expression on my face when Nate would condescend and correct me on set. The unending control was uncomfortable for all involved. They witnessed the tendencies. They felt the pressure and stress I endured. And they did such a great job holding their tongue and staying professional when Nate served as my assistant and manager, but in the end, he still called all the shots.

Chapter 23

BACK AT HOME

When we weren't building my brand, we were home running the two clubs. And while having the other location was an escape for me a few days a week, it was short lived. After a three-year run, we had to close it down. The building we leased was built half underground, with a parking garage above us, and we could not get the building's temperature to regulate above 57 degrees in the winter or control the humidity in the summer. The building owners refused to cover the costs on the solutions we tried, and after spending $200,000 in repairing the electric issues, and adding gas heaters, we realized we would have to cut our losses.

He would call the club daily, sometimes even hourly, while I was working with clients. I would beg him to let me finish work and told him we would talk later. Most days, after the first several calls, which would usually end with me hanging up on him in frustration, I would leave the phone off the hook and leave my cell phone in my office. I wanted to save my clients the constant disruption of the hour that they paid for every time he was slightly irritated with anything, which was all the time. Looking back, I think the club failure in Des Plaines wore on him and his ego, so he became even more difficult to work with. He had some good days here and there, but his bad days were really bad, and increasing in intensity. I could feel my heartbeat in my throat most days, as the stress and anxiety he gave me started to become unbearable.

He was on me all day, every day, with everything I said, every decision I made, and every person I would interact with. I think it became worse because he felt me pulling away and becoming stronger and less tolerant.

My push back was not anything he ever saw before. I fed off his energy. If he was mean, I was mean back. If he was ignoring me, I'd ignore him back. No questions asked. I didn't care how he was feeling. I didn't care if he was sad, suffering, or miserable. All I knew was that my health could no longer handle this relationship. The good he did for me to offset the bad could no longer sustain my nerves.

The new problem was that I was so afraid of pulling the plug because just as he already made me believe that I could not make it without him as a trainer and business owner, he now made me believe my brand could not make it without him. He was too involved. He was managing my social media platforms. I certainly did not have time for that. He was booking and managing my photoshoots, and my sponsorships. He managed my appearances, and my events. He helped run my broadcasts, etc. Even if I could take it over, with training my clients, there was no way I could keep up with all of it. My confidence would falter, and I would just continue on.

Just one month before we officially closed the doors to our Des Plaines location, our best friends, who owned a very popular apparel company called Grunt Style, had opened another business called Alpha Outpost. At dinner one night, they asked Nate if he would run Alpha Outpost as the CEO. I almost did a backflip; I was so excited! That would take Nate out of my Elk Grove location full time, just as I was going back into it full time! I'm not sure, but I think before Nate had a chance to answer, I answered for him! I screamed, "Yes! He would be happy to run your business for you!"

To be perfectly honest, as much stress Nate gave me and as much resentment I had toward him, I did really want to see him doing something that he would enjoy. He did a lot of great things for me. I will never deny that. He wasn't bad all the time. He helped me embrace who I am today, but honestly, it was best for him to get out of the fitness industry. I could see was no longer enjoying what he did. In fact, most of his clients reported that during their session, he would set them up with two different exercises to superset three times, then walk away from them for that entire set. He would show up again for the next series, and then disappear again. This would go on for their entire hour, every session.

Des Plaines closed, Nate was running Alpha Outpost, I was running Elk Grove and my training schedule by myself, as well as my travel and modeling schedule, live broadcasts, and spending time with my kids. Things, once again, became pretty hectic in my life. But despite the packed schedule, I started feeling less stress, that is until the days Nate walked into the building. I would no sooner hear the back door slam than I would immediately tense up. I never knew the mood that would accompany him through those doors. He came in three times per week for my broadcasts and then sometimes at night. And I would feel the entire dynamic and vibe change the minute he walked into the room.

Chapter 24

AN INVITATION

As my manager, Nate was checking my emails and responding to interview and photoshoot requests. It made sense. He was running my social media platforms and managing my events. There was one email, in particular, that caused some issues. The email included an invitation to a high-profile location and event in Washington DC from Luca, a client who I had been training online for about a year.

A year prior, I had been approached via LinkedIn and hired by a hedge fund manager in Chicago. I did some nutrition plans for him via email, and a few phone consultations. He was extremely busy traveling back and forth to New York, as he also owned a business there. During one of our conversations, he mentioned that he was being vetted for an extremely high-profile position that would move him to DC. I congratulated him but did not expand or ask any further questions. My job was to help him with his nutrition plan, not be star struck by his new "celebrity-type" encounter. I was sure that would not be "cool." I took my business and professional career very seriously (and I still do!).

While I was training him, he asked a few times if I had a boyfriend. I had been asked this before, and Nate (in manager role, and not boyfriend role) had always insisted that I stick to my Linda Steele persona—single, footloose, and fancy free. I would, however, wear my old wedding ring as an initial deterrent to those questions. And when asked about it on broadcasts, I would say something along the lines of "I didn't like him so much, but I liked the ring!" It was my own first line of defense.

Nate would always say, and said in this instance, to tell him, "No, I do not have a boyfriend." With that, Luca asked me to meet him for coffee when he was back in Chicago. I declined and told him I did not think that would be appropriate, as I made a rule not to meet my clients on a personal level. He apologized and admitted he might have read into something that was not there. But over the next few months, he pursued me a couple more times. I continued to decline, and he admitted this was strange for him, as he usually has women throwing themselves at him. To be honest, I had never looked him up, so besides his photo on his email profile, I had no idea what he looked like, but I took his word for it.

Luca's nutrition planning package had ended, and he disappeared. About four months later, I received an email notification with a news article in it that said he had gotten that huge job he had mentioned. I was so excited for him because he told me how there was a possibility that he was going to get this position. I emailed him immediately congratulating him, and within minutes, he responded with, "Thank you so much! I would like to invite you to my going away party at my Chicago condo. I will get you details when I have them."

I politely responded, "Yes, that sounds very nice. Please keep me posted."

By this time, Nate and I had not broken up, but we both knew it was only a matter of time. About a week later, I received another email from Luca, which was the one Nate intercepted. Luca let me know that his going away party had changed to his home in New York, but he really wanted to invite me to this high-profile event in DC. He left it up to me.

Wow…just wow! I had never visited DC but always wanted to. I was not going to turn this opportunity down. What happened next is something that I would never have expected. I ran it past Nate, and he thought I would be crazy not to take advantage of that. The problem was that Linda Steele didn't travel alone. She traveled only with her bodyguard, Nate. I had to run this past Luca. He agreed and asked if this bodyguard was my boyfriend. Sticking to my Nate-approved "script," I answered, "No."

One week before we were to leave, Luca Googled me and was a bit concerned about the photos he saw on his computer screen. All those ones that Nate had posted with a lot of skin were peeking into my life again. Luca saw them all, and while he may have been impressed with how I looked, he was more than a little concerned that there would be a problem with the background check needed to attend the event (not exactly sure why a great body that you're willing to show people means you're a criminal, but I digress). He was still fairly new in his position and was not quite sure what to expect if a bikini model was going to be at his side. Although my feelings were hurt, I did understand. He politely asked if we could postpone this trip when he was more comfortable with his surroundings. I agreed, but I assumed our communication would end at that point. To my surprise, it had only just begun.

Chapter 25

A BREATH OF FRESH AIR

About a week after the conversation about the event, Luca sent me a photo from inside the very impressive building in which he worked right before a meeting was about to begin. I was absolutely flabbergasted. It was like I was having an out of body experience. There was this friend (I would say we were somewhat friends by this point), who worked in this building every day for an extremely important man, sending me pictures, just because. Think about that for a minute. When someone asks, "So, did anything cool or unusual happen today?" I could answer that with, "Uh, yeah, actually."

All I could say was, "Wow, that is really so cool! I can't imagine that ever gets old to you."

He responded, "Actually, the first week or so when I would be in meetings, I would find myself daydreaming because, yes, it is surreal and really cool."

Periodically, I would receive another picture or two. And he would always include a nice note, like, "Hi Gorgeous, how is your day going?"

Wow, what a breath of fresh air. A positive man, with positive vibes, doing important things. This was quite different from what I was used to being surrounded with on a daily basis. Nate would wake up in the morning and no matter how nice, sweet, and positive I was being, he was miserable and nasty in return. So, it wasn't a stretch to see how easily I could get mesmerized by this new treatment and attention. Who wouldn't? You're being treated horribly in one way and beautifully in another—which would anyone prefer?

Over the next month or so, these texts that were seemingly random became not so random anymore. They were now daily. We started to get to know each other on another, more personal level. He made it clear that he was not the *home wrecker* type, but I made it clear that Nate and I were done. We had been done for years, at least in my mind. It was just a matter of logistics.

He started back on my workout program and insisted on stopping by my gym one morning to pick up his workout plan. This made me a bit nervous because I was afraid Nate would be there (he still stopped in all the time). I never knew what his reaction would be, but overall, his reactions were pretty shitty. But there was another fear. I was afraid that I was already becoming emotionally attached to Luca. And if he was half as cute in person as he was in his pictures, it was going to be even harder to stay away.

Luca showed up on a Sunday morning on his way from his Chicago condo back to DC. And he was even more handsome than in the photos—*shit!* I spent some time with him going over his program. He asked a lot of questions about my gym and business. He was impressed with all that I had built. He seemed genuinely interested in me and my life. He was one of those types of men that you can tell almost instantly is just a really nice, good man.

I was already reeling with new feelings I hadn't felt in a very long time, so when he kissed me on his way out the door, I nearly fell over from the shock. I knew it was wrong on my part. After all, I had not broken up with Nate yet, so I immediately told myself, "Nope, not attracted to him." I reminded myself that I would have to keep telling myself that.

As soon as he got into his Uber to the airport, he sent me a text that said, "Wow." I wasn't sure what he meant by it, so I asked. His message read, "That kiss. Just Wow." Okay, I realized that I could tell myself anything I wanted, but this guy was going to make my life very complicated. And I knew it. I also knew that he had no idea that Nate and I were still together. We never officially ended it. We were just miserable with each other. *Shit! How did I let this happen? Why did I allow it to get to this point?*

The answers to these questions are clear … now. I allowed it to happen because I had been in a miserable relationship for years. I was longing for someone who would be positive in my life, someone with whom I could have an actual conversation that didn't result in a screaming match. So, when it appeared, even unexpectedly, it felt good—really good. To be welcomed by someone, rather than pushed away and controlled, is admittedly a great feeling.

These once daily texts turned into morning, noon, and night texts. At one point, I was more transparent about my situation with Nate. I started feeling guilty that I had become emotionally attached to Luca and was disrespecting Nate in this way. Luca was not very happy that I wasn't honest from the start, and texted back one day, "Why don't you let me know when you are 100% single." Fair enough. I had that coming. It was weeks before I heard from him again.

I decided I needed to come clean with my emotional affair (let's call it what it was) to Nate. I pulled him aside one day and said to him, "I'm doing something that is very disrespectful to you, and I feel really badly about it."

He looked at me and said, "Go ahead…"

I told him I was having an emotional affair with a client, and that I knew it was dishonest and I felt awful about it. I followed up with, "Sometimes things like this happen when a relationship is failing or if one or the other is not happy, and I think that maybe if we go to counseling, we can figure out why I am doing this."

His response was, "Well, since you are the only one doing anything wrong, you should go. Let me know how it goes."

Well, part of me was upset that he was blaming me, and not taking any of the responsibility himself, but another part of me was thinking, "Damn, is he really going to make this that easy? Okay!"

So, I made my counseling appointment. And it was good. And when I did not fall to my knees at home and beg Nate for forgiveness, Nate decided to come with me for the second appointment, which was pretty uneventful. I don't remember much about it except that the counselor asked to see us each separately, then together, and keep that schedule for a bit until she could get to know us better. Nate was the next up, but his schedule conflicted with the appointment, so he cancelled … and never went back.

I was beginning to feel very stuck again. And this time was even worse because I had such positive feelings and energy when I was talking with Luca. It's like being really thirsty and then having only a sip of water, but the glass is quickly taken away. Suddenly, you're dying for that water. It's the same when you're remembering feelings that have been buried for a long time—once you feel them again, you want to feel them more and more. And I was about to.

The butterflies hit again when I received a text from Luca. It was a picture of the invitation to his organization's Christmas party. No, "Hello, how are you?" message. All he wrote was, "Next year, you are going with me!" I was so happy to hear from him! All those amazing feelings came flooding back in. It was such bad timing though. I was still going to counseling and thought I owed it to Nate to try to make it work. Deep down, I knew I was done with this relationship though. I was so unhappy with him and had been for so long. I just couldn't figure out how I would manage without him. Of course, those were his thoughts in my mind, not my own. But there was a lot that would need to get figured out.

He ran my social media, my website, and anything that helped generate revenue outside of the gym. He helped manage things at home. He even still helped me with the kids. My girls were now grown, but my twins were working for him, so again, the connections and the ties that he created bound us together in entirely too many ways. He had been a constant in their lives for so long. Since they were now teenagers, he was the one who took them for ice cream when boys broke their hearts. He was the one who paid for their prom dresses. He was the one they called when they had a flat tire. There was just so much history between them.

Just as I secretly (but not surprisingly) hoped for, Luca started sending me more text messages again. He could tell that I was not as engaged as I once had been, and this time, I wanted to be completely honest with him from the start. I told him about what was going on between Nate and me. He asked if it would be best that he stay away for a while and I told him, "Yes."

This was not what I wanted at all. I wanted to keep talking to him more than anything else. He made me feel so good at a time when I felt badly far too often. I enjoyed his texts, his compliments about my work ethics, his kind words about the kind of mother I was—I wanted more of all of it. It was like medicine to me. But as requested, he went away again.

Chapter 26

A NIGHT OF TERROR

A few days after New Year's 2018, there was a night where Nate couldn't sleep. This wasn't an odd occurrence. He had been going through a very difficult time that stretched far beyond our issues. He wasn't sleeping, he wasn't eating right anymore. He watched war movies or any movie with blood and gore on TV all night long. It was not a good situation.

On this particular night though, when he couldn't sleep, he came upstairs into my room while I slept (we had not been sleeping in the same bed for about a year now) and went through my phone. He looked at all my messages with Luca since we had started talking a couple of years prior. *Why didn't I delete them?* Well, because he knew that I had been communicating with him here and there as a client and I felt that deleting anything would be sneaky. I didn't want to be sneaky, but sometimes I am too honest for my own good. He went back downstairs and then he called me. His voice was shaken.

I immediately went downstairs. I remember that he was sitting on the floor up against a wall in his bedroom, yelling, "I went through your phone! You are in love with him!"

Nowhere in these text messages had either of us ever said the word, "love," but sometimes it's clear. He said, "I can tell by the way he messages you every day and says all those nice things to you and calls you gorgeous! Every day he tells you to have a good day, tells you he's thinking about you, and then says goodnight! And you eat it up!"

All I could say was, "I'm sorry. I'm sorry." I assured him I was not in love with Luca. But he was not having it.

We continued to scream, yell, and cry together. And before I knew it, my youngest daughter came running into the room asking what was going on. I yelled at her to call 911 because I was worried what might happen next.

Now, while I was very worried about him, there were also a ton of other things running through my brain—I was scared for myself and getting hurt either on purpose or by accident and I was scared for my daughter, who was now witnessing this horrible situation firsthand. There were so many awful and scary things running through my head, I felt like it was spinning out of control. And sadly, this wasn't the first time I had to call the police during an altercation (or when I should have but didn't).

Once Nate heard that she was calling the police, he calmed down. I would not leave his side because I wanted to make sure he was ok. He sat on the floor again, against the wall and told me all the things he was going to tell the police. He was going to tell them I was cheating on him and in love with another man. An emotional affair, in my eyes was cheating. In love? I was not…yet. I just told him that was fine, thinking to myself—*like they would care, but whatever.* I wasn't going to argue. I just wasn't. This was intense as hell as it was.

The police came to the house shortly after. Two were downstairs talking to him, and one was upstairs talking to my daughter and me. They suggested he leave and let the situation diffuse. That needed to happen. I don't know that he would have voluntarily left my home otherwise.

That night my daughter witnessed something that she will never unsee…

My daughter was twenty years old at the time, and she was visibly shaken. No matter what age—young or older—our children are watching us. My daughter had an opportunity to learn something from this, and I hoped that it would be courage and strength of character. I couldn't help but think about when I was nine years old, and I had to call the police to defend my mother, who was in an abusive situation. Now, granted, my stepfather never touched her again, but we did not know it was going to turn out that way.

My daughter and I had tears flowing down our wet cheeks, more in disbelief and shock than anything else, as we watched him leave down my long driveway. We both were in awe, flooded with every emotion a person can feel. We didn't say much to each other. There was not much to say. It was now 3:00 a.m. and I had to be at work to open the gym at 5:00 a.m., so we simply hugged each other and went to bed.

I don't think I actually fell asleep (who could possibly sleep after that?), but at 4:00 a.m., my phone rang. It was the police. They told me that unless I didn't mind him coming back home, I would need to come in and sign a statement of what had just occurred. I woke my daughter up and we got in the car to drive to the station. We had had no sleep and just encountered one of the most devastating moments of our lives. And now, we had to write a detailed statement, reliving it all.

I am not sure how I managed, but somehow, I made it to work at about 5:30 a.m. By this time, I was sobbing. It all finally hit me … hard. As soon as I walked in, one of my members and good friends spotted me and saw the look of distraught on my face. He immediately took me by the arm and walked me right into my office. I sobbed uncontrollably into a gym towel—all the emotions, all the negativity, all the fear that had been bottled up for years came out in those moments. I tried to tell him what I just encountered, but I am not sure what actually came out of my mouth.

He insisted I go home and take a few days off, but I refused. I had a couple of new clients starting that day, and one at 7:00 a.m., so I had to be there. My work ethic was something that I would never allow anyone to change. Besides, what was I going to do at home other than be more miserable? I tried to rest in the back room in between clients, but I could only keep up this tough exterior until about noon. I had to go home. I could not stop crying, and I could not tell anyone why. The emotional floodgates had opened.

I made it home okay and told my daughters we were having a family meeting that night when they got home from work. They knew Nate was not there, and they knew why, but I told them they could not tell anyone. I am not sure why, but I felt the need to save his reputation in any way that I could. As always, *Linda the protector* was in action.

When my daughters came by that night, my youngest daughter and I explained all the details. One of my daughters was so happy that I was finally out of what she referred to as, "an abusive relationship." I was a little confused, I am not kidding, because I saw it like that at times, but I guess it just became normal to me. And I definitely, and foolishly, thought my girls didn't pick up on it. Well, of course, they picked up on it! As I've said before, my girls are extremely smart and intuitive. I couldn't hide shit from them if I tried. One of my daughters asked if I would ever take him back. And before I could open my mouth, the "little one" (she'll always be my baby) answered for me—"Absolutely not! He will never live in this house again! It is him or me!"

I did not need her to answer for me, but I am glad she did. I was so used to taking him back and feeling sorry for him over the years that I was not sure I trusted myself. Now, she set the limits, and it was up to me to listen to what she was saying. I appreciated that more than I can say.

I decided to take the next few days off to try to get my bearings back. I felt as if I was floating aimlessly, not exactly sure which way to go or what to do next. That's one of the many problems with this type of over encompassing relationship—your partner works his way into becoming your anchor—holding you down with enormously heavy chains until you can barely move or breath. It is literally like you are drowning in your own life. So, when that pull is ripped apart, yes, there is freedom, but there is also no direction when you no longer have that center of gravity. Admittedly, that's a scary place.

I did not tell most of my clients why I took time off, but there was one couple who I was honest with when I called them to cancel their sessions the next day. When I started to share my story, I started to cry. Immediately, they told me they were coming over. They arrived at my house soon thereafter, and I began to tell them what had happened. Before I got very far, the phone rang, and it was Nate. He called me and told me he was coming home. I apologized and told him he could not come to my home. I told him I couldn't have him here after what had happened. I reminded him that my youngest daughter still lived in the house, and I was not comfortable with him being there.

He was furious. I stuck to my guns, and it absolutely infuriated him. He was firmly talking as quietly as he possibly could, but my clients could still hear him through the phone. They heard him tell me it was my fault this happened. It was all my fault, and he would never forgive me for ruining his life. As he was talking, I was just sobbing. I didn't say anything, other than, "I'm sorry."

When I hung up the phone, this couple sat on my couch in awe. They could not believe the words they heard him say. Muffled or not, they got the gist of it—this was an extremely dysfunctional relationship. They merely said, "Please tell us you do not believe him. Please tell us you know you are doing the right thing."

I cried and cried and told them I didn't know if I could live without him because I was scared that I could not do it on my own. Then they asked me, "Specifically, what are you afraid you can't do?"

I still can't believe this was my response—"He fixes everything here. What if the sump pump goes out? I don't know what I would do."

The client offered her husband and said, "He knows how to fix a sump pump. Don't worry."

And in the weirdest, most unexplainable way, I felt secure. Now, this had nothing to do with the pump and everything to do with my own mental state. In retrospect, it's clear to me that it is what happens when you've endured that kind of mental and emotional abuse from a very young age and for so many years after. Your thinking becomes warped, your concerns are overexaggerated for the simple things, yet underexaggerated for the more serious issues. And while you're in this state, you simply can't decipher between the two.

So, for the next several days, I looked like I saw a ghost. And I felt so much guilt. I cried day and night. No matter how you slice it, this was a bad situation. I know why people stray, but I couldn't believe I did it, and I did take blame for it landing Nate where he was.

About three nights after the incident, as I was in the fetal position on the couch crying, I heard a notification from my phone. It was Luca. He texted, "It is harder to stay away than I thought it was going to be. How are things at home?"

I couldn't even answer at first. Again, this man was so incredibly sweet and lifted my spirits every day. But when I first saw that text, I was torn. It was so nice to hear from him, as always, and so nice to hear that he was thinking about me, but at the same time, my guilt was suffocating me. *Guilt for what though? Guilt for liking that someone finally spoke to me nicely? Guilt that someone made me feel good about myself? Guilt that someone finally made me feel smart again? Worthy?* I deserve someone who made me feel this way, damn it! My daughter was right. I was leaving this relationship.

I texted back telling him that things became worse, and I that I was devastated, but it is being managed. He asked if there was anything he could do to help and asked exactly what happened. I told him I would rather not talk about it and that it was just going to take time for me to get through it. I thanked him for his concern. He respectfully backed off and told me he was coming to Chicago over the weekend and asked if I would like to meet him for dinner. I never responded.

I was in no condition to meet him. I was a mess. I could not stop crying. This went on all day and all night. I did go back to work after taking the rest of the week off. But that didn't stop me from crying all day, every day … for 35 days straight. Every day, my trainers would walk in the building and peek in my door to see how I was. Chances were, if I was in my office, I had my face buried in a gym towel, crying. I was so scared to be alone. I had never been alone up to this point. For decades I was surrounded with others—unfortunately, usually by toxic people though. I simply knew nothing else.

I was so distraught thinking about what happened that night. What if someone had been seriously hurt? I couldn't help but think that I may have had the closest brush with death. In these heated outbursts when emotions are at their highest, anything can go wrong. Unfortunately, in some cases they do.

One of my trainers walked me off the gym floor more than once because it looked so unprofessional with the owner of the gym training clients with tears running down her face. My clients were just trying to be supportive. They stopped asking questions, and knew that when I was ready, I would open up.

Not long after, Nate asked again, but I still would not let him come back to my house. Because he knew me well, he was good at getting me to feel sorry for him. He was so good at letting me feel like I owed it to him. He was so good at letting me think I couldn't do it without him. Honestly, I thank God every day that my daughter was living there, and I could not let him back in for her sake. She did not want him there. And I would honor my daughter's wishes before I did anything else.

I am afraid to admit that if she had not been there, I would have let him back in. Nate had spent years employing interrogation techniques, psychological warfare, and other nasty mind tricks to foreign enemies … and to me. And the impacts were devastating. And I still felt sorry for the man that I had once loved deeply. I was not strong enough. Yet.

He found a temporary place to live in San Antonio, with our best friends. These were the same friends who had offered him a job to manage their store. Now, they offered him a place to stay (once again, rescuing me). They had no idea what they were doing for me. They thought they were doing it for him, but I benefited from it more than he did. I finally had some relief and less guilt—he had a safe place to stay. I didn't have to worry about that. Plus, being so far, I knew he couldn't just pop into the gym anymore … or my home.

Luca checked in with me about once every few weeks to see my progress. He was starting to worry about me because any progress I did have was extremely slow. Anytime we "spoke," it was through texting because I was still crying a lot and told him I'd rather not get on a call. He offered his help, but he didn't know how exactly I was struggling because I never told him the story about that night. I only told him that I was scared. He continually asked for clarification on that. I finally told him I was scared to be alone. And then he continually asked for clarification on that too. He now discovered that I may not have been 100% honest about my situation with Nate. He realized that he was more involved in my home life than I had led on. Luca had made it clear a long time ago that he was not a homewrecker. And I had made it clear that I was done with Nate. Neither of us lied, but somehow here we were.

Nate continued to remind me of all the things he did for me and how if it weren't for him, I'd be nothing. He reminded me of the work he did on my house, how he helped raise my kids, and how he taught me my career. He continued to remind me how I ruined his life … even from San Antonio. I went from never locking my doors at home, day or night, for twenty years to installing a security system, changing the locks, and making sure my gun was loaded and next to my bed. This was not a great way to live, but it was the necessary next step in my transformation.

MODELING, TRIPS, AND FEAR

My modeling career and social media influencing had started picking up in a big way in 2017. I was already booked out for the entire first quarter of 2018 with photo shoots, speaking events, and even an Oscar gifting suite debut. I was co-hosting LA Talk radio, and other online stations, and traveling to Minnesota, Vegas, LA, and Long Beach, California regularly. These trips were scheduled before our lives were completely turned upside down, but I did not want to cancel and seem flaky or be unable to fulfill my obligations. My name was important to me, and so was my business and brand. My commitment was unwavering—a good thing, right? Well, kind of. The problem was I still did not feel like I could do any of it without him. And so, the door was opened once again … a door which he happily walked back through.

The first trip planned was to Vegas. I was a special guest invited to a big annual party that was hosted by Grunt Style. That party was followed up by my very first topless shoot at Red Rocks, just outside of Vegas. A second shoot was scheduled with another photographer for the infamous shot in my red steampunk outfit.

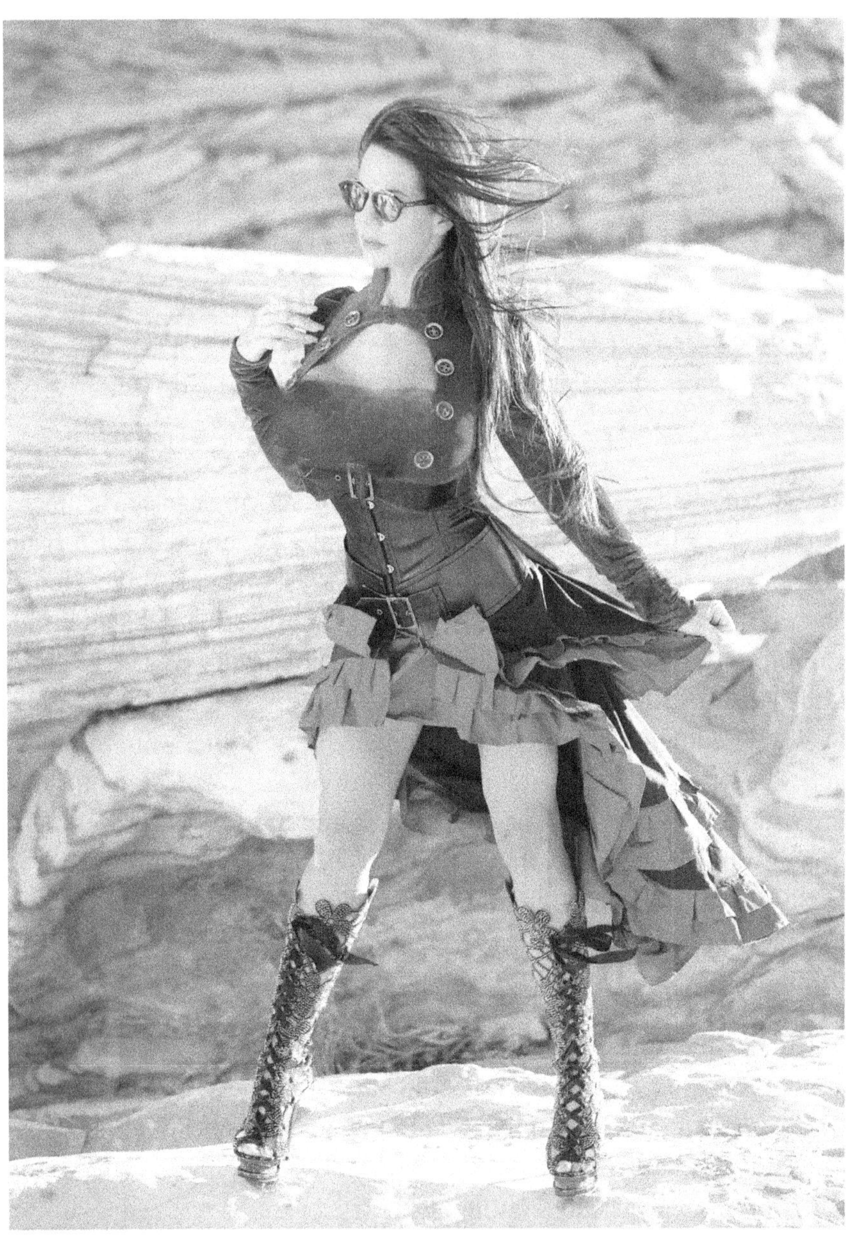

Photo by Victor Broden Photography

The morning after our first night in Vegas.
Infamous shot in my red steampunk outfit

Nate and I met at O'Hare airport, after he flew in from Texas. This was a few weeks after he had gotten settled in with our friends in San Antonio, and the first time we saw each other since that dreadful night. We hugged hello, and within five minutes got into a huge argument because he left me at security, as I was sorting out an issue. I had to get through the entire airport to the furthest terminal, and, of course, the last gate in my six-inch heels, with my two carry-ons. Now, this does not seem like a big deal today, because I travel alone all the time, but back then, I had never had to touch a single piece of luggage when Nate was around. I walked freely anywhere I went if he was with me. And for that I give him credit—he acted the part of a gentleman in public and even in the privacy of our own home … at times.

When I arrived at the gate, he was standing there, chit chatting with a man. They both looked at me and I gave Nate a stare that would scare the shit out of anyone. The man said something to him that I was not able to hear, but I was pretty sure he was saying prayers for him. I ignored him the entire flight, but if I got an opportunity, I was as mean as I could possibly be. Once we arrived in Vegas, he tried to talk to me, and I completely blew up at him. Yep, he managed to pull the CRAZY out of me … all the time. He was not saying anything to rectify the situation or to apologize to me, but he was definitely trying to cool me down. And I was not having it. I started looking for flights to go home right then and there. I was seriously just about to book a flight home that departed in an hour but remembered all the people counting on me. I remembered all the commitments I had in the next few days, and I just couldn't leave.

Mutual friends picked us up at the airport, and they could immediately see that things were not good. They were trying not to pry, but also trying to make everything seem normal for the sake of all of us in that stress-filled car. Unfortunately, it didn't work. I was fuming.

I wish I could say the rest of the trip went smoothly, but I can't. While it was very productive, it was very rough. I had committed myself to the Grunt Style party, Shot Show, meetings, and two photo shoots, so I had to go through with it. And I am not sorry I did, but the costs were high. Those were a scary few days for me based on the way we were both behaving. I was afraid of what might happen, but I also found that I could no longer "play nice" for his or other people's sakes. I was over it … but still scared of what that attitude might lead to.

Within minutes of us arriving at the hotel, Nate became very angry. He was clearly angry about us breaking up and was afraid I would never take him back. I tried to calm him down without giving any false hope. And this scene went on for hours … to no avail. Honestly, again, I was starting to be afraid of what might happen next based on our escalating anger. I'm no psychologist, but it seemed like the behavior of a very desperate person.

At this, I contacted Victor, my photographer for the first shoot, and asked him to be on standby. I briefly explained some things to him, but there was no way I could get in front of a camera and put on a smile and act like everything was all good. I can put up a front here and there, but I am not an actress, which was exactly what that would call for—acting my ass off.

I am not sure how, but I managed to calm him down just enough to get us ready to attend the pre-party for the event at Grunt Style that night. We arrived at the club, went directly to our table, and met with friends, including the friends who picked us up at the airport. I immediately apologized to them for my behavior earlier that day. One of them completely understood (I think my situation reminded her somewhat of her own) and she was very supportive.

When we arrived back at the hotel that night, Nate was absolutely shitfaced. He fell asleep (aka passed out) pretty quickly. Thank God. No interaction. I was not drinking that night, as I knew I had to be in tip top shape for my first photoshoot of the trip, at sunrise the next morning. This was my very first topless shoot ever, and although I was pretty sure nobody would be looking at the bags under my eyes, I still wanted to make sure I looked my best. I alerted my photographer and let him know we were all good to go.

We made it to the shoot just before sunrise. Nate had always been the greatest assistant in helping with wardrobe (or lack thereof) and overall getting from point A to point B, on time, without forgetting any details. On the other hand, he also excelled at making me a nervous wreck during this time. *Give and take, right?* My anxiety was always through the roof, with this loose cannon type of behavior. He made mountains out of mole hills every chance he could and put such unnecessary stress on me. And it wasn't just me. Everyone was always on high alert when Nate was in the area.

It was like a breath of fresh air when I arrived at this shoot, despite the fact that I felt Nate did everything in his power to make me think he was going to go off the deep end at any minute and embarrass the fuck out of me. My photographer was very familiar with his behavior, and that actually gave me some comfort along with my embarrassment. I didn't have to explain anything. He already knew every time I arrived at a shoot exactly how I was feeling. Because of this, he did everything he could to negate my uneasiness and make me feel as relaxed and comfortable as possible.

The shoot went even better than expected. It was possibly the best shoot to this date! A photographer will make or break the tone of the shoot. This guy had a lot to overcome that day with Nate and with making me comfortable on my first topless shoot, while dealing with colder, windier weather than was forecasted. We shot at two different locations, and as the day went on, the temperatures warmed up and we fell into our groove. It is such a joy to work with absolute pros that go above and beyond to make the magic happen.

We ended up with a six-hour shoot before we closed up shop and started getting ready for the Grunt Style party that night. I was expected to

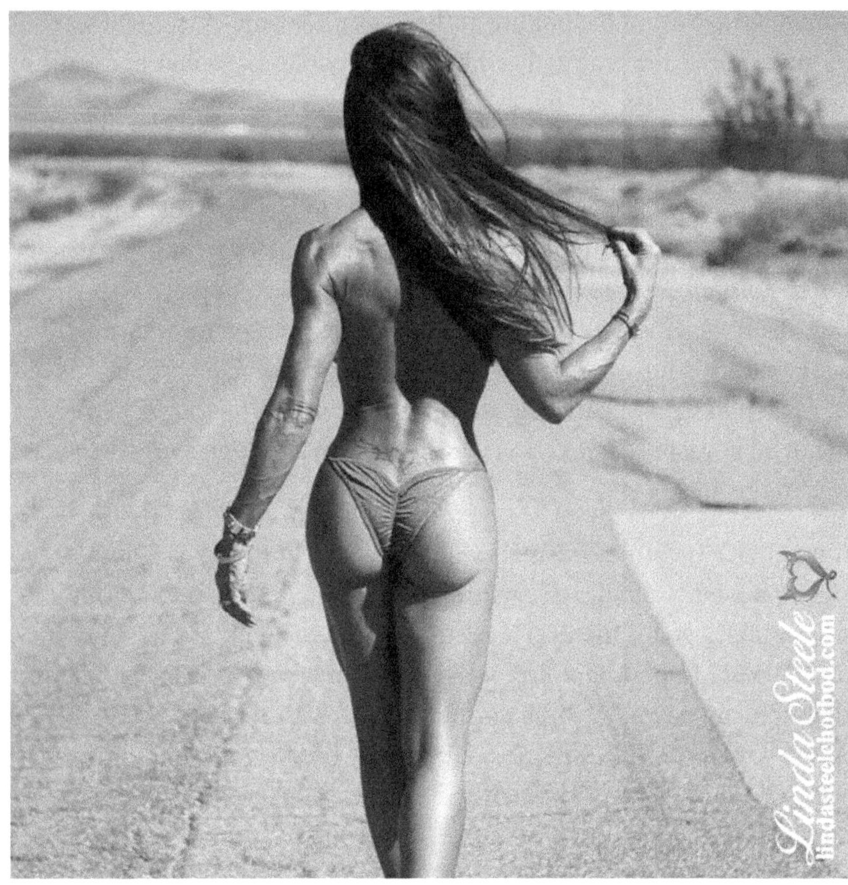

Photo by Victor Broden Photography
My first topless photoshoot
Dry Lake Bed, Las Vegas, NV

work the crowd at this party and put on my best smile, but as always, I felt unnecessary stress being added to my evening because of Nate. That was just what we did together. It was our dynamic. If I wasn't walking on eggshells every minute of the day, he felt like he was losing control.

Despite all this, I couldn't wait for the party! This party was a really big deal. Grunt Style had just spent two million dollars on a Super Bowl ad that was going to début in front of all these VIPs that night. Our friend, the owner, had shown it to me before. Plus, I was in LA watching it being filmed live, and it was all so exciting! As their best friends, it was great to see it all come together for them.

Most of the people at the party knew me or knew of me. I spent time mingling and enjoyed every minute of it. Nate was nowhere to be found, which was very unusual for me, as he was not only my boyfriend all these years, but he was also my bodyguard. Within a short period of time, he was hammered again, and picked a fight with me while I was talking to two gentlemen about social media, the party, and other mundane topics. He appeared to be extremely jealous suddenly, when in the past, he would display me around like his piece of property, like a kindergartener on "show and tell" day.

I left the party quickly after that. I could easily see which direction this was heading, and it wasn't good. One difference was that I was more concerned for him embarrassing himself than embarrassing me for the first time in our relationship. But I also didn't want him to distract from our friend's big night that was all unfolding in front of potential investors and other VIPs. Leaving was the best option. Nate, of course, followed me and tormented me all the way back to the hotel saying the most awful, disrespectful, disgusting things. I tried my best to just ignore him.

We made it back to the hotel and he went to his bed and passed out while I washed up and prepared for my shoot the next day. Nate woke up right as I fell asleep and started another scene. This time, he was as close to outraged as you could get. He was furious with how I was talking to men at the party. He called me every name in the book. According to him, I was a "whore and a piece of shit." This went on for quite a while. I just kept my mouth closed while he screamed. I thought my life may be at risk once again, but at some point, he stopped. I don't remember much else about this painful night.

The next morning, I had promised to meet with a fan, and a couple of other social media influencers. I went down to the lobby a bit early because I wanted to look for other flights home. I felt like I needed to get myself out of this situation. As much as I didn't want to disappoint anyone, there was no way I could go through with the rest of my weekend responsibilities—not in this frame of mind.

I couldn't find any flight that wouldn't cost me thousands of dollars, so, I stayed. I followed through with my obligations. I met with everyone I needed to meet with that morning and even made it to my shoot that afternoon. I guess Nate was on strike that day, so he did not help me at all with any of my commitments. I had always counted on him to help with packing and remembering all the wardrobe details for the shoots. It wasn't that I couldn't do it myself, I just didn't know I had to leave time for all of it. I would usually only give myself time to get ready, so having to do everything to prepare affected my routine. We ran late, and once again, this made me even more nervous than just his presence and the uncertainty of when the next blow up would be.

We drove to the shoot location in the same car. Nate was very friendly with the photographer Sean Kirk, and his wonderful wife/assistant Jean. I was pleasantly surprised—actually, I was shocked. I just never knew what to expect out of him, especially after a night like the one before. Somehow, the shoot went smoothly—better than I expected, as it was the first time I was shooting with this photographer. I ended up being glad that I didn't cancel on him. To this day, these photos are some of my favorites.

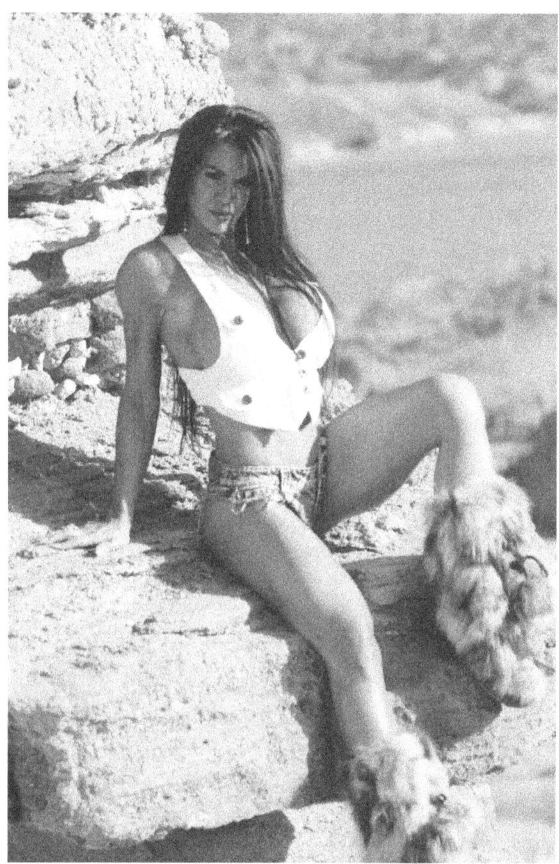

Photo by Images by SMK, Colorado River,
Las Vegas, Nevada

I made it home after that trip and had one week before my next event at the Leigh Steinberg gifting suite in Minnesota for Super Bowl weekend. The trip was fairly uneventful, even with Nate there. It just so happened to also be the weekend I was launching my topless section of my website. This was a nerve-wracking time for me. I had never released photos like this before and I started to get cold feet. But it was too late—there were already hundreds of people signed up for this unveiling of my boobs! Needless to say, it went very well, and I am not sorry.

Chapter 28

A NEW RELATIONSHIP

Nate went back to San Antonio where he was living, and I went on running my gym and being a mom. I did the best I could, but I found myself still feeling very sad, scared, and guilty a lot of the time. Sad that life as I knew it was about to change drastically, scared that I could not do anything on my own, and guilty for having the emotional affair and for leaving Nate in such disarray. He acted like his life without me was doomed. He also continued to make me feel like I could never make it without him. As much as I wanted to break away from him, I had no idea how to manage my website, my social media, my events, and my photoshoots—my entire brand—without him. Nor did I have the time to learn. I had a business to run and clients to service and three daughters to be there for. It was a constant sense of uneasiness.

Somewhere around mid-February, I received a text from Luca. "I'm coming to town this weekend and I would love to see you. Are you up for it? I know you had a pretty rough start to your year, and I was hoping things have settled down a bit."

I talked to my daughters and mother about this, and they all thought I should go. Even though I did not feel ready to be myself yet, I agreed. I told him I was only available Friday night so he wouldn't expect the entire weekend. I met him at the restaurant, and it was so strange to actually be on a date. This was a man who made me feel like a million bucks weekly, sometimes daily.

It was the weekend after Valentine's Day, but he still bought me a few gifts. I was absolutely not expecting gifts, and I felt awful for not having one for him. We had a great dinner in the city and went back to his hotel after to watch a movie. He let me choose and I said, "Pitch Perfect II." It was one of my favorite movies, but to this day, I cannot believe he asked me out on a second date after that! When the movie ended, he asked me to stay the night, and I declined. I wanted to go slow this time. I knew I could really fall for him. And all the way home, I thought about seeing him again. The next day I went to work, and I called him to thank him for dinner. I told him I was available that night too, but he had already booked a flight back home.

He flew in again a few weekends later and we spent another day together. We talked daily now, and he eventually asked a lot of questions about my brand and what I do besides owning the gym. He was familiar with Instagram models and so forth, as his ex was big on social media, but he was not sure what my end game was. Was it just to be popular? Was I able to monetize this somehow? So, I let him in on how it worked and told him that since I had a website, I was able to advertise to a ton of people. And that they now know I offer something for sale on my website.

"What would that be?" he asked, skeptically.

"I have a subscription section. It's for members only, where they pay a monthly subscription for exclusive photos," I responded.

He looked at me. "Huh. What kind of *exclusive* photos do you offer for this paid subscription?" he asked softly, "Nude photos?"

I replied, "No, not nude, just topless."

There was a long pause, then he asked all the right questions, "Is this something you want to do? Is this something you *have* to do? Are you getting paid a lot of money for this?"

I was truthful about it—I felt like I could be with him, "The truth is, I've been asked for years to do this, and I've always said no. I have a mom and I have daughters and I need to take them into consideration."

I explained that my social media fans were getting restless, and this was clearly the next step, but it wasn't until I started working with European companies when I realized how different Americans view topless photos than the way Europeans view them. "The Europeans look at the woman's body like a work of art," I explained, "and that is how I am looking at it as well."

Then I showed him the amount that I made in the first month from my website sales. He was impressed but told me matter-of-factly that he would have given me that much money *not* to start doing those types of photos. But this was my choice, and my life, and I was not sorry.

I really started to like him, and the feeling was mutual, but I had several more events coming up that I had committed to. This time, I was going to LA, Beverly Hills, Long Beach, Malibu, and the surrounding areas. This was a ten-day trip full of speaking events, photoshoots, and appearances. Luca was a little confused why I was going to be traveling with Nate, as my manager/assistant, when we had broken up. He never acted insecure about it, but he did seem concerned. I had opened up about my Vegas trip to him, and he was trying to be supportive, but offered other options that I turned down. I just knew it was going to be a really busy ten days, and I had never done any of these things without Nate. I was not comfortable doing it any other way.

It was a very productive ten days, and everything about it was great. Even Nate had a good attitude the entire time. As I snuck around and spoke to Luca here and there, assuring him things were going well, I had the added security of feeling like my life was not at risk. Coincidentally, it was during this trip that I also snuck the last phone call to solidify my life insurance policy for my kids in case of accidental death. It was just always in the back of my head. As supportive as Luca could be (and we

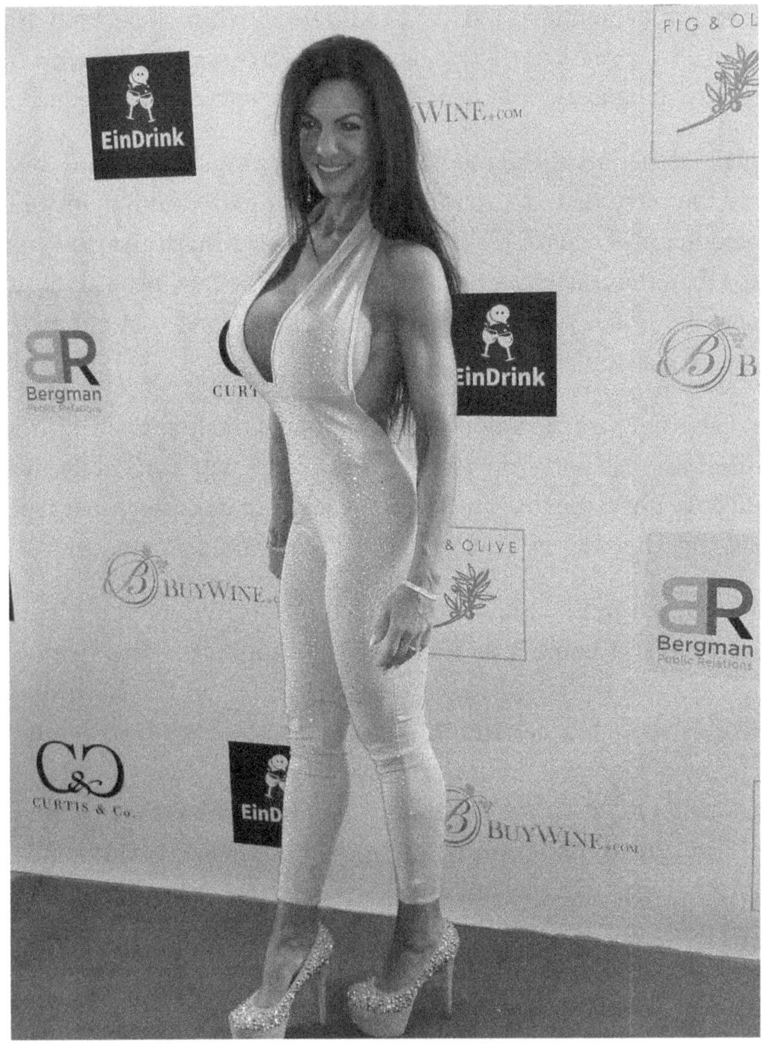

Doris Bergman Gifting Suite
LA 10-Day Trip of photo shoots, events and appearances,
and red carpet interviews

were not exclusive at this time), I could tell he was getting a little anxious for this trip to be over. I am sure he was wondering if Nate and I were going to get back together, but as far as I was concerned, that was never going to happen.

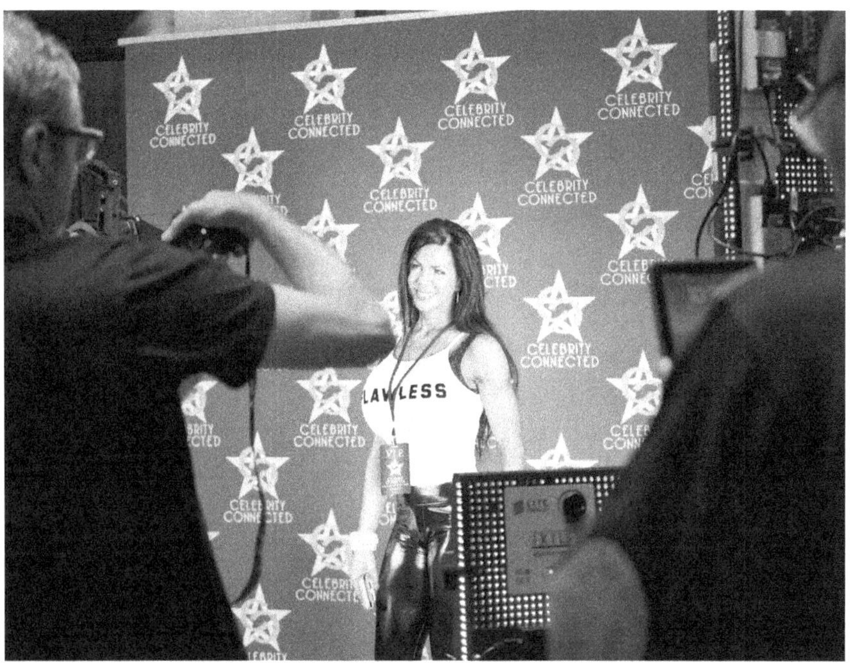

Gifting Suite in LA
LA 10-day Trip of Photo Shoots, events, appearances and red carpet interviews

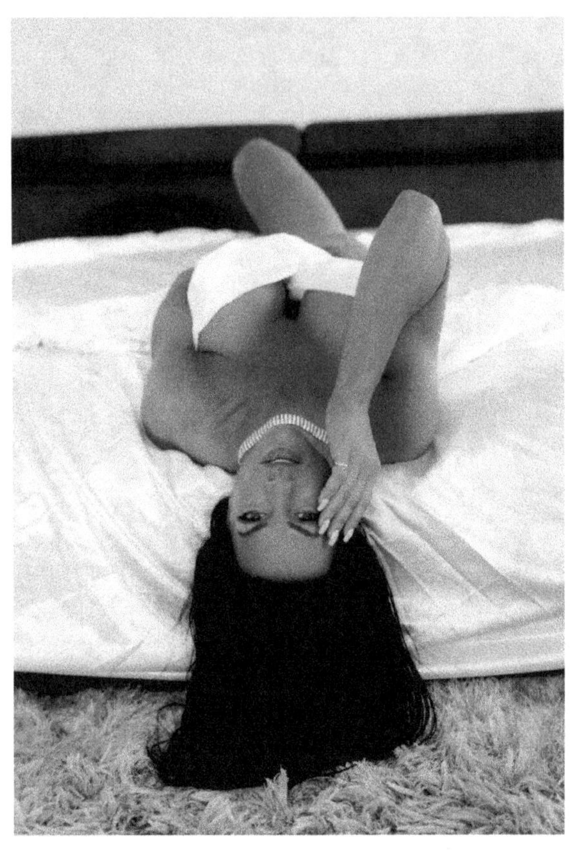

LA 10-Day Trip of photo shoots, events and appearances,
and red carpet interviews
Photo by Images of Bliss

Chapter 29

STEPPING INTO
MY OWN ... AND SMILING

Luca came to Chicago once more over the next month, and we continued to talk every day. At the end of April, we met in Orlando for the weekend. I was selling a condo there and he accompanied me, in case I needed him and for us to spend some time together. That weekend was a turning point. On Sunday, before we left, he asked in his "Luca" way if I wanted to be exclusive. He said, "I have decided that I am not going to date anyone while I am with you, and I would appreciate it if you would be honest with me if you are going to continue to date people."

It was rare to hear such honesty from a man, at least in my experience. I told him I would do the same, even though I had a few concerns. Let's just say I had a couple of "loose ends" I needed to tie up if this is the case (people I had been "talking to" during this time). But mostly I wondered if I really wanted to jump right back into a serious relationship. I had not really "dated" since before I was married, but I did not want to let this guy go. He was so kind and encouraging and caring. I couldn't imagine why I would want to date anyone else. So, we took our relationship to the next level. We started seeing each other regularly, either every weekend or every other. We mostly met in New York or Chicago, and always had the best time together.

I was still seeing my counselor, and she kept asking me specifically what I was afraid of as far as ending things with Nate. When I had to stop and think about it, I realized one of the scariest things for me was to do a photoshoot without him. So, I charged ahead and did one. In May, I crossed a huge bridge that I thought I'd never do alone. I booked and planned my first photoshoot without Nate as my assistant. I chose a photographer I was comfortable with. He knew my whole story and situation, so he promised me it would be perfect.

I had asked Luca if I could use his house in Lake Tahoe for the shoot, and he was excited to be able to do that for me. Not only was he happy to help, but he had a driver pick me up at the airport, and his property manager there when I arrived to make sure I knew my way around. My photographer arrived and things went better than perfect! It was one of the best photoshoots I had ever had. My most favorite shots came out of that shoot. You could see it in my face—I was happy, smiling, natural, relaxed, *and* I was having fun!

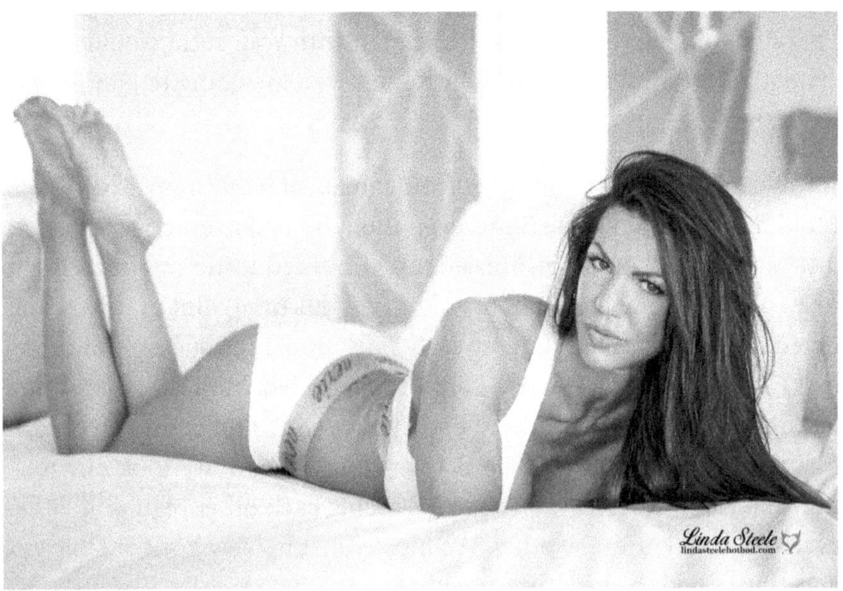

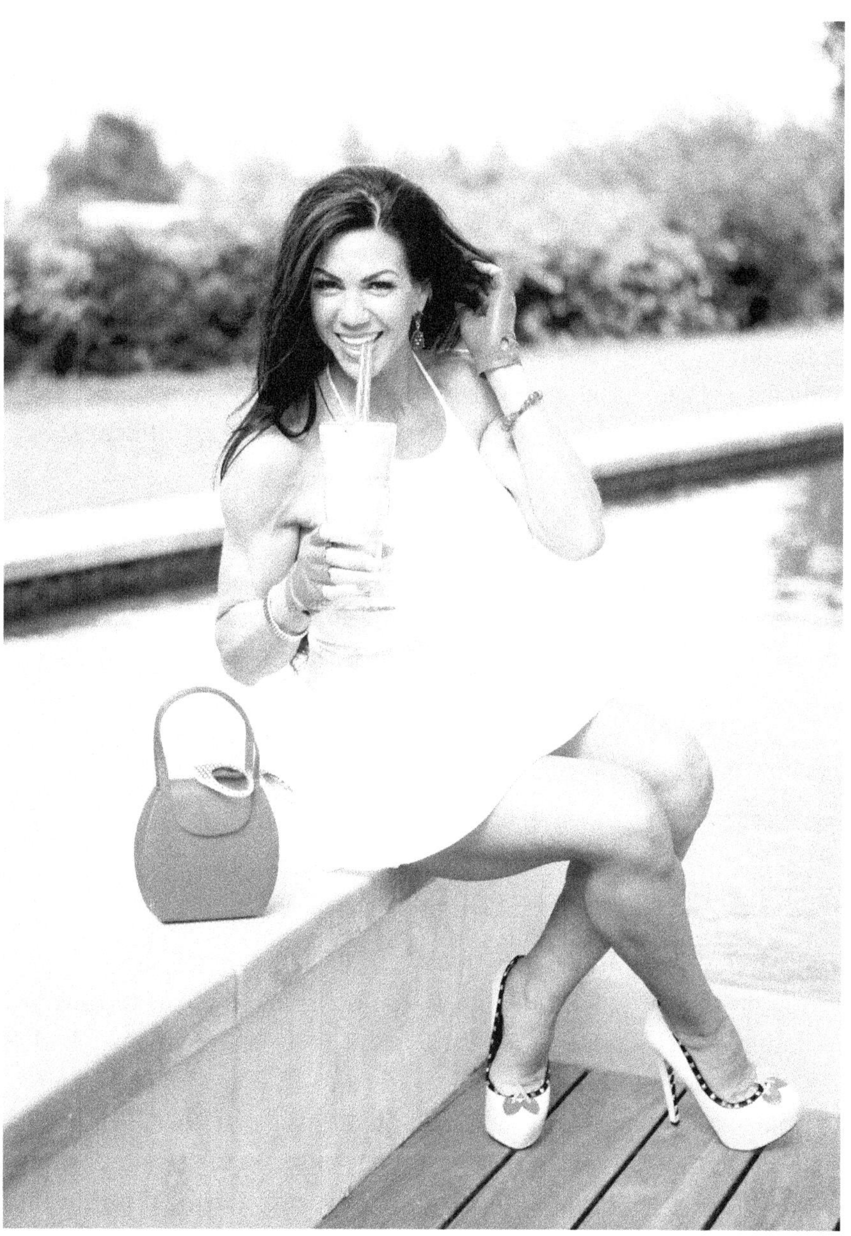

Photo by Victor Broden Photography
My first solo photoshoot feeling relaxed and
Having fun! Lake Tahoe home

With the help of so many amazing friends and colleagues, and of course, Luca, it took me five months to 100% break away from him. But all these people helped me not get overwhelmed by taking over a small aspect of my life or business, and before I knew it, they each handed it back over to me. And I was able to handle it … on my own. I cannot describe how liberating it was—the moment that I discovered I could handle it all. It was gradual, but when I did, and I looked back, it was absolutely the most empowering moment I could ever remember in my life. I was free of the unnecessary, daily stress that Nate put on me. I realized I was just as smart as I remember being before I met him. I was making decisions once again without having to ask permission. I got my confidence back. I started smiling again…all day, every day!

Luca and I spent the weekend in California. He brought me to the greatest places and introduced me to some friends. We saw some landmarks and had a great time. He knew I was a huge hockey fan for the last several years, since I started going to the Chicago Blackhawks games in 2011, so as a surprise, he bought us tickets to the Stanley Cup in Vegas. We took a road trip to see the Knights play and it was amazing! We had the best seats in the house. In fact, when we went into the owner's box (he was friends with some of the owners), I wanted to go back to our seats because they were so much better! I was so impressed and felt so spoiled. I just couldn't believe he did this all for me.

Tuesday morning, it was time for me to fly back to Chicago. We were laying on the bed, sweet talking before he dropped me at the airport, and I told him I was *not* ready to go home. He asked me to stay. And as much as I wanted to (and I really wanted to), I knew I had a business to get back to. I had clients to manage and a gym that I owned. So, I left that day, but we did meet in California the following weekend. It was so great to always have something to look forward to during this time. My life went from being miserable to being so exciting! My mom used to tell me all the time how nice it was to see me smile again. She had not seen me happy in years—her daughter was having the time of her life!

With these pleasant days came havoc, however. Nate was not going anywhere easy or quickly. He knew I started up a relationship with Luca and was furious. I felt he was not going to make this easy on me. Unfortunately, he was back living in my area and made his presence known. He would show up at my gym unannounced … yet again. He continued to approach me even if I was with clients just to say something degrading, disrespectful, or intimidating. Once, I was at the front desk signing up new members and he walked in and started interrogating me right in front of them—it was so embarrassing. I texted him a few times telling him he was not allowed to just walk in unannounced. It didn't matter.

On Mother's Day in 2018, I had my mom, daughters, and sister and her family over. I was standing in my kitchen having one of the best holidays I could remember in a long time. Then, I received a text from Luca, asking if a particular phone number was familiar to me. I had never seen it before in my life. He said, "this person claims to have incriminating evidence against you."

I had no idea who it could be and told him so. He continued to send me screenshots of the conversation along with a picture of three people in bed together. One of the women had my exact tattoo on her lower back where mine is. He asked me, "Is this your tattoo?"

I responded, "Yes, it is, but that is not me. I have never been in bed with another woman, nor have I ever been in a threesome."

He said, "I believe you. I think I know your character by now, but if this isn't you, you should get to the bottom of it, so this photo doesn't show up someday and hurt you."

I was absolutely furious! I may not have had proof, but there was only one person who had reason to do this. I could even tell by the text itself. Only one person in my life had ruined every holiday, every year, since the day we started dating, why stop now? I was having the time of my life, and the best, most relaxing holiday. I have no idea what phone he was using, a throw away phone for sure, but I don't even care.

I exploded to my family as these texts were coming through. They were not aware of the depth of my break-up with Nate. In fact, they were wondering if I was going to fold and get back together with him. I decided it was time to tell them exactly what happened that awful night in January to put their minds at ease. They felt so bad that I had waited so long. They would have been there for me. And I knew that, I just couldn't talk about it. Every time I talked about it, I had to relive it. I just wasn't ready to do it again.

Luca felt it would be best not to accuse anyone of anything at that point. Nothing good could come out of it, which would only make matters worse. It went against my character and was against everything I knew and everything I believed in, but I was able to keep it in … even that same night when Nate stopped by my house unexpectedly.

I did not let him in the house. I stepped out onto the doorstep and sat with him to talk a bit. The entire time, I was trying not to lose my shit over what had just happened. I know him better than he knows himself, and he was trying to feel me out for sure. It appeared he was trying to see if I was mad or startled. He even said that with the two of us being so well known in the community, there would be people who would try to ruin us, individually. He said that people are jealous and vindictive, so I should watch out for people like that in my life. I just shook my head. It didn't matter what words came out of his mouth at that point. He finally left, and I went to bed.

For a day or so, I once again looked like I saw a ghost. I was mad, sad, frustrated, and scared. Was he going to try to ruin me? When would he stop tormenting me? Texting and communication with Luca didn't seem any different, but I was sure it was in the back of his head that I could possibly be lying to him. This could be the end of things for me. I was positive that he was not about to deal with this type of drama in his life—not at his level or in his position.

The following day, my friend, who stood by my side always, refusing to let me fail, asked me what the hell was going on with me once again? He thought I seemed at ease for a little bit. Why the setback? I have never been known for hiding my feelings, so I showed him the picture and the text that Luca received. He was absolutely shocked. And then he did for me what I thought was impossible. Somewhere on the internet he found the original picture of the threesome that was sent, where it was very clear that it was not me.

I immediately contacted Luca and told him I was going to forward him these originals. He told me he was happy for my sake that I had them to clear my name if ever needed, but he believed me and saw no reason to see them himself.

"Besides," he said, "Your legs are much nicer than the woman's legs in the picture."

While that was nice to hear, it was nicer to know that he truly trusted me. It was a relief to know that he truly believed in me. And on top of all of that, he could even make me smile at a time like this. This was starting to feel like a healthy relationship, and it made me happy and at the same time sad—after all these years, I didn't know what that was like.

Around that same time, Luca had been looking to buy a condo in California. He had been working with a realtor, and within a few weeks, found something he loved. That day was pretty funny, as we had been out with my nephew and his girlfriend drinking mimosas before looking at properties. I am not a big drinker and never have been, so it didn't take much for me to be completely shit-faced. Then, we walked into this gorgeous $5 million home on the water that looked like something from the movies, and I stood in the doorway, doing a slow 180 turn with my head. I looked at the realtor and said, "We'll take it!" We still talk about how hard we all laughed!

By the end of May, he closed on this gorgeous condo, and we started playing house. He let me decorate it and fill every cabinet and wall with anything I wanted. We went together to pick out most of the furniture, but he pretty much handed me the reins and told me to have fun. I tried not to make myself too comfortable there, but he only referred to it as *ours*. He was more than a little bummed when I moved my weekend clothes into a different bedroom, rather than the master. He wanted us to share everything. But I knew he was used to living alone all these years, and I didn't want to cramp his style.

We were there almost every weekend, and I was living my best life for sure. Things at home started becoming a little difficult though. My kids and mom were super excited to see me smile for the first time in years, but I was still trying to run a business. I had a gym, employees, and clients to tend to. And I was so torn. I had obligations, but this lifestyle was very easy to get used to. I also honestly felt that with everything I had been through, I needed to have some fun. I needed to laugh and be carefree a bit.

At the beginning of June, Luca's sister and her husband and co-workers were coming in from out of the country. He was so excited about me meeting them, but I was surprised that he wanted to introduce me to them. He mentioned that his family had not met a girlfriend in years, and I suddenly felt some pressure sneaking into the relationship. This was when I started to realize that I was being very guarded. I was actually searching for the red flags I was so used to seeing. I had walls up around me and would not allow myself to get too close to him.

I thought maybe this was a temporary situation. He had dated many famous people in the past, and I never thought he would be trying to settle in with just one woman (and truth be told, especially if that woman was me – there were all those old doubts and insecurities coming back). Based on his high profile, I just did not feel worthy. There was nothing he ever did to make me feel unworthy, just the opposite, in fact, but this just seemed like a fairytale, and I was waiting for the coach to turn back into the pumpkin. Still, I tried to push past it. He had done nothing to make me feel this way. It was me, and I knew it. And I truly loved being with him.

So, I met the family. We spent the weekend all together, and it was one laugh and one excitement after another. I was pinching myself. My life was perfect. And I had never, ever felt that way before.

Chapter 30

LOVE LANGUAGE

Back home, I was approached by someone who wanted to buy my gym. It was strange because it was not for sale. I was not interested and almost offended, actually. The prospective buyer had been around and noticed that I was only half into it anymore, so he thought it might be a good time to unload it. After my being offended passed, I decided to sleep on it. After all, I had been torn in two for a while then, with my heart and smiles in California and my work there. So, I thought, "Well, why not?" Selling the gym would allow me to continue with this lifestyle, to a degree. I could still train my clients and run my website business to make money. I talked it over with my kids and made the decision. I was going to move forward with the sale!

Not long after, Luca came to Chicago, and it was that visit when we finally exchanged "I love yous." I had been thinking about it for a while, but just wasn't sure how I was going to tell him that I had fallen in love with him. I was sure that he was not in love with me (again, totally on me, not him). I had to be honest though. It was very unnatural for me *not to* say it, and when we talked about it, he told me it was very unnatural for him *to* say it. He had a Russian heritage—not typically the warmest people. So, growing up, he didn't hear or say it very often at all. He assured me that he would get better at it and from that day on, he said it often.

This was also around the time when I stopped updating my website regularly. Because he was high profile, I knew it was best for me to keep a low profile. My members will tell you exactly the timeline on that. They felt it, and the numbers started dropping off. I lost about 50% of my monthly revenue once I stopped updating regularly.

My web guy who had been helping me run my social media was very concerned that I was throwing this revenue stream away. He reminded me that if this guy goes away, it will be very difficult to start from scratch and reminded me how hard I worked to get this momentum going. He was right. But I didn't listen.

"What are his intentions? I mean, is he planning on marrying you?" he asked.

I just looked at him having no idea what to say. We hadn't talked about marriage.

"If you let this revenue drop, and he breaks up with you, does he plan to cover your loss?"

Again, I didn't have an answer. These were great questions that I did not even feel entitled to know. Yes, I thought about the cost of letting my hard work fade away, but for once in my life, I was living in the moment and having a ball! My weekends were epic! Trips to DC, New York, Lake Tahoe, Miami, and California, staying in penthouses and homes worth millions, driving in expensive, luxurious cars.

But above all the glitz and glimmer, above all the fancy restaurants and clubs, what I loved the most was finally being with a man who appreciated me for my intelligence, drive, and determination. Luca told me how impressed he was with me and nearly everything I did. It took 48 years for a man to tell me what I needed to hear to make me feel worthy. It took 48 years for a man to show me he cared about me and what I wanted. I had a man fulfilling my needs for once. Finally, a man discovered my "Love Language," and I never even had to tell him what it was!

Every day I smiled. Every day I had reason to love my life. Every day I knew that a man saw the good in me. We had a long-distance relationship that was more fulfilling to me than any relationship I ever had. Yet, as far as I had come, I ended up in the same place in some respects, namely with Nate. He just couldn't let me be. One weekend, while I was away in California, he called my daughter and asked if she could bring him my dog (he had bought it for me one year before), as it gave him some comfort. She asked me for my approval, and I said it was okay because I felt so bad for him. Two weeks later, my dog was dead. He was hit by a car. I still do not know all the details, and he never told me what really happened. But I never wanted to speak to him again —not even for an explanation.

Little did I know that my new take on life—all the smiles and laughter, all the fun and trips—was about to come to a screeching halt.

Little did I know that some of the people I love the most were going to go through some very challenging times.

Little did I know that the decision to sell my business would come back to haunt me.

Little did I know that I would have much bigger things to worry about, like my boyfriend fighting a newly detected illness.

Chapter 31

TRYING TIMES

The fun and the smiles and the laughs came to a screeching halt. He, of course, gave me an out. He did not want me to have to change my life to deal with a sick man. He and I both knew that the next six months were going to be very difficult and at times awful. It did not take me long to think about doing the right thing. I told him that when I said, "I love you," it was not the fun lifestyle I loved. I was not going to leave him at a time like this. He had no family here, and only work friends and superficial friends.

Within a week of diagnosis, he had surgery, and we continued on the path of recovery. Medical treatments started and went on every two weeks for about six months. I tried to be there as much as I could to take care of him, making soup and chili and whatever comfort food he wanted. But then I'd have to get back home to work and to my obligations there.

My mom had just had hip replacement surgery and needed constant care. My sister helped a ton though, which freed me up to go back and forth to Luca. But I soon noticed that my mom was having some medical issues separate from the surgery. One night, my sister called as she was leaving the rehab facility, "Okay, I just left mom. She is doing great. She was almost asleep when I left her so you should rest assured all is good. No need to worry about her."

I was so relieved to hear that. I had not had time to see her that day. I was able to stay at the gym and get caught up and prepare for my next very long day. As soon as I hung up with my sister, my phone rang. It was my mom. "Hi, mom."

My mom screamed into the phone, "Linda, get me out of this hell hole!" She continued on with how uncomfortable the pillows are, how annoying the nurses were, how bad the food was, and anything else she could complain about.

To say this was a tough time for me would be a huge understatement. My boyfriend was just recovering from surgery, my mom was having some medical issues, and my dog was just hit by a car and killed. When these personal trials and tribulations weigh you down, you can't possibly make clear decisions, including for your business.

The gym sale had been taking forever. But we finally we made an agreement—if you can even call it that—I basically signed the worst deal I could have signed. I wasn't thinking straight, and I didn't have an attorney, which made room for the buyer and his attorney to take full advantage of my situation. Had I known the type of man who was buying my gym, I never would have done it. He completely changed the atmosphere, the dynamic, and the vibe. Everyone started to feel like a guest instead of like family, how I had treated them. There is still talk about how rude, arrogant, unfriendly, and unreasonable he was.

In addition to how he treated the members, less than one year into our agreement, he stole some of my equipment and sold it, and then broke the lease, leaving me responsible for another year—double whammy there. That was when he stopped paying me for the remainder of what he owed me, which was well over $100,000. And just when I thought he was done fucking me over, he stole more of my equipment and brought it to another location to start his own gym. Another hurdle for me to overcome in my life at the hands of a shitty man.

Once the sale was finally over, I continued to be with Luca as much as possible, while juggling time with my kids, making sure my mom was ok, and catching up with friends and family. It was actually a really great time for me on one side, but a really sad time for me as I watched him struggle in the horrible aftermath of his medical treatments.

Once the treatments were over, we tried to get things back on track. We started traveling together again, I learned how to ski, and we celebrated our first Christmas together. Just after Christmas, we went on a two-week trip to Europe, where he brought me to meet his mom. This was a pretty big deal, as he had not introduced anyone to his mom in fifteen years. Meeting her and other members of the family was a bit nerve wracking. I knew they were high class and sophisticated, but they were also so much fun!

From the minute I met them, we hit it off! They remembered to speak English and if they didn't, Luca made sure they were reminded—even if they were having a conversation amongst themselves. I told him, "No worries, they were not even talking to me."

He said, "I don't care, you should never wonder if someone is talking *about* you."

That was just him—always was courteous. And then it changed. After several more trips together, his entire attitude was different. He said that since he realized how short life is and that he could die at any time, he would rather not have the responsibilities that come with a relationship. I was so confused. *What the hell just happened?* It was at that time that he *texted* me, "After seeing how you took care of me while I was sick, I wanted to marry you. Now, I don't want to even be in a relationship with you or anyone. I'm sorry."

That was quite a blow. I wasn't sure how to even respond. And it was via a text! Just weeks before, he had written me the sweetest Valentine's Day letter, and now, he wanted to break up. And only one week before, he had come to Chicago and took me, my mom, and the kids to dinner. He wanted to thank them for holding down the fort with my gym and taking it over while I was taking care of him when he was sick. He told the kids that as a "Thank you," he wanted to take them all, including the boyfriends, to *our* condo in California to go explore the city and take a trip to Napa. He called it the "Steele Team 8 Trip."

I am not sure what changed overnight. He had described our relationship as "effortless." I was so confused, but I gave him what he wanted. We were done, and he got very cold after that. I am guessing he wanted me to beg. Well, I didn't. It was probably the easiest breakup he ever had. My ego wouldn't allow it to go any other way.

During the breakup, he made it clear that he wanted me to act like the condo was mine and come visit anytime I wanted. I did actually visit it a couple of times when he wasn't there, but it was much harder than I thought it would be. For one, when you looked out the balcony, you could see the hospital where he was initially diagnosed. But more than that, we managed to make so many great memories there. It was a time in my life when someone finally made me feel wanted and appreciated. Appreciated and smart. Smart and worthy. All of it. I couldn't stand to be there anymore.

Six weeks after our break-up, a close friend talked me into seeing him once again in DC. He insisted that I was better than being broken up with over text and then Facetime. He was right. I was. I deserved more, damn it. I called Luca out of the blue, in the middle of the workday, and he picked up immediately. After some small talk, I asked him if we could have dinner together. I made it clear it was not an attempt to get back together, but more of a proper, "Goodbye"—closure, if you will.

He sounded a little taken back and asked, "Do you think we are ready to see each other just yet?"

I answered, "Well, yes, I thought we were trying to remain friends. You've mentioned the connection we have with one another being there for each other during our darkest times. Friends are allowed to spend time together."

He responded with, "Well, sounds like you're taking this better than I am. I am still struggling with our breakup. I'm seeing a counselor, and I'm not sleeping at night. I still have a lot on my mind, and I am a little shocked you are over this so fast."

I explained that it was not that I was over it, but he broke up with me, and I really had no choice but to move forward. I wondered how he thought I should be responding. *Mixed signals for sure.* He didn't really have an answer for me, but he asked if I could come later in the week. I did, and I spent the entire weekend with him.

He met me at the cab when I arrived at his place, and I got the biggest hug and kiss. He held my hand all the way to his room, and we talked and laughed and swung arms like two teenagers. It was like things never ended. We sat and talked for about an hour or so. During that time, I was able to figure out that he was definitely over me. We still had a great weekend together though. He held my hand as we walked and even at the dinner tables. He even moved his chair closer to mine several times at restaurants. He still acted like a complete gentleman with my doors and chairs. When it came to the bedroom, he held me so tight all night long, but not once did he try to be intimate with me, and I was relieved.

The morning I was leaving DC to come back to Chicago, we had breakfast together before he went off to work. During breakfast, he mentioned once again that our breakup might be the biggest mistake he ever made. He mentioned I was one of only three women in his life who got embedded into his heart. He did not hint that he wanted to get back together, but he wanted me to know how important I had been to him.

I walked him to work like I always did on Mondays before leaving to go back to Chicago. When we got to "our" corner where he would kiss me and go off to work, we turned to each other. We both knew this was going to be the last time we would be at this corner together. He grabbed my face with both hands and said, "What we have is too special to lose completely."

I responded with, "We were friends first. You will always be my friend." My response didn't even go with his, but it was what came out of my mouth.

We kissed, and we walked in opposite directions. I remember looking back once. I am not sure if he ever did. I didn't have the answers but am smart enough to know that even great love stories die unexplainably sometimes.

Chapter 32

MY FREEDOM TOUR

Here I was, 48 years old and single for the first time since I could remember. We could go all the way back to junior high, and I can tell you I *always* had a boyfriend. I had no idea how to date. I didn't even know where to start. And, on top of it, I was not my friendly self … to say the least. In fact, I was unhappy, short with people, and disengaged. I was lonely and very distracted. I had a lot of unanswered questions rolling around in my head. Everyone around me started to try to boost me up, telling me I was Linda friggin' Steele and that I could have anyone I wanted, anytime I wanted. But the simple fact was I didn't have anyone, and it felt wrong.

After months of refusing to get on a dating app called Bumble, a co-worker of mine finally forced me. One night, he would not let me go home until I built a profile. He actually built it for me once I provided him with five of my favorite pictures. I just had a really bad attitude about the whole thing, but somehow, I had a coffee date by the next morning! I had conversations going with several men at once, but this one met me for coffee. We had a great time together and even had a second date. He ghosted me shortly after that. I am not sure what happened, and I don't care. It was shitty, and there's no excuse for that.

The next few months, from an outsider's perspective, probably appeared to be a ton of fun for me while I played at this dating game. Besides Bumble, I just so happened to run into one of the "loose ends" I had to tie up when Luca and I had decided to become exclusive a couple years before. He was a marine pilot, and we had only gone out a few times, but each time was a great experience. One day, we both happened to have a layover in the same city at the same time while I was on my way to Vegas for a photoshoot. Let's just say we made the best use of our time there, and what happens (on the way to) Vegas, stays there. I even managed to check something off my bucket list that I didn't even realize I had!

During my "Freedom Tour," as I began to call it, I managed to go on a few dates with some really nice guys, but I just wasn't finding anyone with whom I wanted to be in a long-term relationship. I didn't want to fall in love. I didn't want to commit. I think subconsciously I wanted to force myself to be alone until I was comfortable with it. At the same time, I was not meeting the right guy. Great guys, but not *my guy*. But I think that my type was still a developing concept at this point. Nonetheless, it was the start of my "Freedom Tour," and it was absolutely epic. I have no regrets. Not one.

And one by one, I was weeding them out on Bumble. I went on several dates, but my co-workers and friends could not keep up with who was who, so my friend made a list on the white board at work to keep them all straight. The board was filled with nicknames to make it easier to remember. For instance, the Marine pilot's nickname was "Top Gun." The one who ghosted me happened to be a retired NHL player, so his nickname was "Hat Trick." Some names were fun and funny, some just to the point.

"Bag o Donuts," was one of the first, and we had a great time! We met in Miami, but he had been pursuing me for years back while I was with Nate. I posted on my social media that I was in Miami. My mom had come with me on that trip to stay at my friend's penthouse, and

I received an email from him saying he was in Miami and would love to meet for lunch. I was pretty vague, but I told him my mother and I would be at the Fontainebleau for lunch, and he was more than welcome to meet me in the lobby, so we could get a selfie or something. And he took me up on it! I let my mom know that we might have to stop in the lobby for a few minutes and she was totally fine with it. So, I emailed him back asking for a picture, so I knew who to look for. *Wow, just wow!* I was not expecting a hottie like him! Even my mother was impressed!

He met us in the lobby, we talked a bit and took a few pictures. We mentioned we were hungry, and so was he, so we all had a three-hour lunch together outside by the ocean. The conversation never went dull, not even for a minute. As we were wrapping up, he asked me, and then my mom if it would be ok to take us to dinner too. My mom backed out and insisted we go together alone instead. *Thanks mom! She's the best wingman ever!*

After dinner we went to his Spanish style, 12-bedroom mansion on the canal. This place was enormous and beautiful! After the tour of the house, we stood by the pool and kissed. A lot. There was immediate chemistry. He asked me to stay the night, and I declined. *Was it tempting? Very.* Now, I realized I was old enough and I did not need permission for anything, but I didn't want him to get the wrong idea about me.

He came to visit me in Chicago the following weekend, and we were so excited to see each other again—giddy actually! And nervous too. I hadn't felt like that since Luca. But the butterflies would have to wait since he was in the middle of a business deal going bad, three hours after he arrived. There were texting wars going on with a partner from one of his businesses, who emptied the business bank account. His life was also being threatened by this guy and a Mexican Mafia drug lord. Needless to say, he was *quite* distracted. *I swear, you can't make this shit up.*

The bad partner and drug lord completely ruined what could have been the start of a fun relationship with a guy I was crushing on so hard! *I want a re-do!*

I told a very close friend of mine this story and he asked me, "Uh, Linda, you don't see any red flags here?"

My answer was, "No! He was a great kisser, and I am crushing on him!"

Back on Bumble…
I was ghosted on a Saturday by the guy I referred to as, "Hat Trick." He and I had planned on going out that night. Obviously, that didn't happen because he stopped responding to texts. I had no problem staying home, and actually got comfortable on my backyard furniture. I laid on my couch enjoying the weather and jumped back on my phone to start swiping on the app. I started messaging a man who looked interesting, and it turned out we were both free that night. I got decked out as usual, and we met at a restaurant a few hours later.

We completely hit it off! We met again in the city the following weekend and had dinner on the rooftop of Trump Tower with friends of his. Another great night for weather in Chicago. The fireworks were a nice touch, so was the bougie club, Three Dots and a Dash, we went to afterwards. We were so smitten that we booked a trip to Cabo three days later. His nickname on the board was "Cabo."

We met in the gorgeous Mexican town, as he was coming from a business trip in Vegas. He was a commercial real estate developer, so it made sense that we stayed at one of his developments in Cabo. He showed me all around and we drove to the most private beaches. Consequently, I checked more things off my bucket list.

We had great conversations on this trip, but once we arrived home, he sent me a very long text telling me how we were perfect for each other in so many ways, but he wanted a simple life, with no kids. He knew that I was very close to my kids and spent a ton of time with them. I was glad he broke it off quickly. I was not attached yet. Just excited that I might have had a boyfriend who had a place in Cabo!

Back on Bumble…
I committed to a weekend date after hours of phone conversation with a really nice guy. This man shows up 80 pounds heavier than his pictures reflected. We're going to call him "Hot Rod," due to the boner he had the entire time we were together. I let him know in advance there would be no funny business, as I don't do that on the first date. Thank God he was the nice man I thought he was because I put myself in a very dangerous situation that night. He drove three hours to meet me, so I agreed to stay with him. This was not a good idea on so many levels and, although it turned out okay, I will never make the same mistake again.

Back on Bumble…
I decided to go on a solo trip to Miami—a little alone time was exactly what I needed. Shortly after I arrived, I put on a great bikini, went down to the pool, picked out my chair, and oiled up. No sooner had I put my sunglasses on and started to lay back on my chair, when I heard from across the pool, "Hey Linda! Want a drink?"

I sat up in my chair, and across the pool I saw a beautiful man standing with a bottle of champagne and two champagne glasses. Now, I barely drink alcohol, but after three seconds to digest what he asked me, I said, "Sure!"

I stared at him as he walked around the pool to where I was. Once he got to me, I asked him, "Did you call me by my name?"

He said, "Yes. I asked the pool attendant who you were!"

We drank for the next several hours and even made friends with another couple at the pool. He asked me to come to his place to watch the Democratic debates, as we both had interest in politics. He was a secret service agent, so we both had great stories to exchange. He cooked me dinner and we had a really nice time. We were discussing the condos and he wanted to see one of the penthouses, so I brought him up to the friend's penthouse I was staying in. I showed him around, and then he hugged me and left. I washed up and climbed into bed.

My phone went off with a text from him that said, "Would you have been surprised if I kissed you?"

I responded, "I was surprised that you didn't."

He followed with, "I'll be right back up."

Checked off another thing on that bucket list.

The next several men I dated made it to the board with names like "Dancing King" and "DC 2.0," but they all had something that I simply could not overlook in someone I'd want to build a long-term relationship with.

Right around now, my kids were starting to get worried about me and the decisions I was making. A bit of a role reversal hiccup in our lives. They were happy I was having fun, but they did not like that I was venturing out with "strangers" who I barely knew. My mom, well, I think she was just living life vicariously through me.

Back on Bumble…
Back home. Met and went on a couple more dates with different men. This round was a pretty good one actually! They were all nice looking and one or two were even consistent with the communication. But it was the last one who actually made his way into my heart. His name on the board was "Touchdown."

Touchdown and I weren't even supposed to meet. He happened to be on his way to O'Hare Airport from up north, which put him in my 50-mile radius set on my app profile. We matched and I messaged him right away. He was gorgeous in his photos (not that that always means anything). He was about to board a flight to London with his family, but said we'd meet up as soon as he arrived home in ten days.

For someone who was traveling abroad, I was surprised how consistent he was with the communication. He messaged every morning with "Good morning" photos during the day of his trip and said goodnight every night. That was very unusual from the other men on this site, and it grabbed my attention. We went through the *getting to know you* questions and comments during this time, and the day after he arrived home, we met.

I was floored by how handsome he was. I mean, I was more attracted to him than any other man I met during this dating extravaganza. In fact, I couldn't remember being that attracted to another man in decades! We sat at this restaurant for several hours talking about so many things. He was a total gentleman and asked if he could kiss me at the end of the night. The kiss was almost too good to be true. I knew I had to see him again!

After he walked me to my car and went to his, he came back just as I was pulling away, and said, "Wait! We need to get a selfie!" *It was a great excuse for another kiss!* We made plans for that next Friday, which was only four days later, but it seemed like eternity. It was just the time I needed to tie up loose ends and clear off that board!

Chapter 33

FULL CIRCLE

ouchdown and I spent the next several weekends together. This was exactly the relationship that I was comfortable with, work until 8:00 or 9:00 at night, no one waiting for me to get home, seeing my friends and family when I want to, and then great quality time with my boyfriend on the weekends. And quality time it definitely was. We traveled, we worked out together, we loved doing house projects together, he taught me how to golf, we went to the firing range together, he showed me the appreciation of watching football—we just had fun with everything we did! We became best friends.

We started traveling some weekends to visit his boys, and it felt like I had the same lifestyle I had with Luca, which is what I missed. All my needs were being met, and it seemed like his were too. Until the moment when he realized that my social media presence was not going to be easy for him to deal with.

I attended an event and was unable to invite him. There was a video that started circulating of me getting attention at the event and when I saw him the next day, he had an attitude and did and said things to me that he shouldn't have. That night, in the most non-confrontational way, I mentioned it to him, and he did apologize. At the time, that was good enough for me. Not losing my shit over it was completely out of character for me, but I was evolving too. The weekend turned out to be great for him and his son, so I am not sorry I didn't blow up.

As time went on during this relationship, there were times when it felt like he was passive aggressively trying to make me insecure. I am not an insecure woman, so that is hard to do, which is why I wasn't sure exactly what he was trying to accomplish by saying the things he did. He showed me time and time again how much he loved me. I tried to overlook things because I knew, by this time, no one is perfect, and sometimes we have to take the bad with the good (as long as it is not unhealthy or harmful to us).

I was truly grateful for all the wonderful things he did for me and felt lucky to have him in my life. He was kind, he was thoughtful, he was very helpful, and he loved me. He got me through some tough times— times I wouldn't have wanted to endure without him. But I was under the impression that he had unfinished business with previous relation- ships, and it was wearing on me. This was one of the things that made me feel like I was never going to be enough for his needs. There were many times I felt this way over the course of our relationship.

I often felt defeated trying to give him all he needed. When I would bring my reasoning to his attention, I didn't feel the validation that I expected. He was glued to his phone, constantly texting others, and it didn't matter if we were at a romantic dinner, in bed together, or relaxing on the couch with one another. He seemed distracted and it made me feel like I was not his number one priority. It was hurtful, and although I mentioned it to him, the behavior continued.

I started to wonder if he was doing these things on purpose. I thought there's no way that he could do the same thing over and over again when I was so transparent about my feelings, unless he was trying to get a rise out of me. It seemed extremely disrespectful, and that is some- thing I knew all too well, unfortunately. I knew exactly what to look for since I had been trying to escape disrespectful men my entire life.

After almost two years of feeling disrespected on and off, and consequently breaking up here and there, I remembered the key that I tended to forget in relationships—I was the only one in charge of how I was going to feel every day. Nobody is in charge of me but me. So, I had to do something about it.

I had to end a relationship with a man who I loved because I could not trust him with my own feelings. I had to. I had been working with a counselor for years on getting my self-worth in order and identifying when I was being disrespected. I was no longer a minor, I was no longer a dependent, I was not stuck in a business with someone. I had no excuse to ignore my mental state. Bottom line, I was a grown ass, independent woman, who made my own decisions, made my own money, and quite frankly, would rather be alone than have my feelings hurt by someone whom I cared deeply about.

This was now another man I was in love with who didn't seem to love me the same way. I asked for what I thought were the basics. That's all it would have taken to keep me with him. My worth must be set by me. Always. I knew I couldn't count on another man to define it, even one I was hoping to marry.

I was continuing to struggle with the amount of time I had gone through life waiting in line for my needs to be met, while I sat with empathy and compassion for my partners and their struggles. I was no longer willing to sacrifice my happiness for someone else's, but I also understood that it was all a part of the growth I needed to go through. Sometimes, there just are no shortcuts in this thing called life.

I was finally content with being alone. I was finally able to realize that being alone feels better than feeling sad and hurt. I spent far too many years being unhappy, irritable, and depressed in relationships. I wouldn't do that anymore. I wanted to be happy again, and I truly was. But had I not forced myself to do it—to be alone for a period of time—I would have never known. It was empowering.

Chapter 34

A NEW CHAPTER

Back on bumble? No, I was definitely not up for that. Instead, I took the following year to focus on my own goals and accomplishments, such as writing a book. Being alone was something that I had not experienced in true fashion and it's something that I'd always wanted to prove (to myself) that I could do. Feeling alone definitely felt better than having my heart shattered into a million pieces. Making my own decisions without having to run them past another person felt empowering.

I did date a bit here and there over the next year, but just for some companionship and fun—nothing that I was going to put any effort into. I didn't feel as if I was hurting anyone or misleading anyone—they weren't looking for anything serious either. We had fun together, traveled together, had great dinners together—it was nice. At the time, I felt like we were simply filling the void in each other's lives. This period of time also gave me a rare opportunity to take a look within. I was trying to go on with my life and find a way to clear all the negative thoughts of men I had been carrying around for nearly my whole life.

For months, I did not hear from Touchdown. He was done. I was done. I got it. However, after several months of no contact, he reached back out to me. He told me that there were a few things about me (and my persona) that made him very insecure. He came forward, not with excuses or unauthentic apologies for his unwanted behavior (that always made me feel second best), but with logical and honest explanations that he hoped I would try to understand. I hadn't ever seen this side of him, and it quickly caught my attention. The way he made himself vulnerable allowed me to entertain an important perspective that I had overlooked before.

As he explained, instead of telling me he was uncomfortable with something, he would do things that he knew irritated me—things that would obviously hurt my feelings or make me feel disrespected. This made him look like a huge asshole in my eyes. He knew at times he had been out of line, but he struggled with how to be honest about how he was feeling for fear that it might make him look weak (being an asshole seems to always better than being weak in a man's eyes!).

You see, when he first met me, I was Linda Steele doing Linda Steele things. Traveling alone, doing topless photo shoots, interacting with fans, and all that went along with it. Yes, he knew this going into it but didn't realize the other side of it—that I would also be getting random phone calls from fans from all over the world at all hours of the night, receiving dick pics from strangers, reading disgusting and disrespectful comments on social media, and so much more. My social media presence and interaction with the fans was something that he had never had to deal with. He's a protector by nature and had difficulty not being able to interfere, but I had told him he needed to take a backseat, and this was "part of the territory."

He had known what he signed up for, but when the reality hit, he did not like watching men treat me like an object due to the photos on social media and my website. He knew a much different side of me, and often told me, "You're better than that." And although I know my worth, my persona/brand was a source of income that I didn't want to give up. And I didn't think I should have to. He never *told me* what to do or what not to do, but he suggested that *I didn't have to* and that made me feel like they were one in the same. Since I hate being told what to do, especially by a man, his tactic clearly did not work in his favor.

Through his explanations and vulnerability, though, this past behavior started making sense to me. But my trust issues were stronger than any explanation (no matter how logical it was). Back then, I had told him the things he did that bothered me, and he did them anyway. Could it really have been that he was doing those things because it was his way of communicating for the lack of respect he was feeling? I was not going to be fooled, so I was not going to put myself in a position to find out.

This was a true growth period for me. The single life was allowing me to spend a lot of time with friends. And it just so happens that I have a number of male friends. I've always considered myself very lucky for that, as I get a great male perspective on things. I expected my male friends to tell me, "Yeah, fuck that guy, he shouldn't tell you what to do and he shouldn't behave the way he does." But to my surprise, they didn't. They understood that Touchdown's actions were that of man trying to hold it together, as he was constantly fighting his natural instincts to protect, but also let me be me.

These friends of mine who had enough balls to give advice (solicited or not), would say things to me like, "Hold on, this guy is okay with you having *male* friends and you got rid of him?" They'd tell me, "Your standards are unrealistic." I also heard one say, "It takes a different level of security to date a woman like you." But my favorite might have been, "Steele, just because you're a total dime piece and you got a nice rack doesn't mean you can treat men that way." *Wow! Good talk!*

You know how when enough people tell you the same thing over and over and then it just clicks? It took me a very long time and a lot of convincing to realize that perhaps if I was asking someone else to change something about themselves, I could also *maybe* look within myself, too. I had been so hell-bent on not allowing anyone to disrespect me and not putting up with anyone's shit that my rules and standards became very rigid. I started thinking how this might possibly interfere with *ever* having a solid, stable relationship. Did my past relationships dictate my future ones by molding me into someone whose barriers made me impenetrable? Would my heart ever be open enough again to let someone in?

This period of time when I was really looking within and trying to find the right balance between being empathetic and putting my foot down made my youngest daughter question my sanity. She heard me making excuses for, and being empathetic toward, a man who she once heard me complain about on a regular basis. But I started understanding some of the things that he did, and the reasons behind them.

She was shocked and confused, as she was not used to seeing me "soft" like this. One day, she told me, "I don't know what's going on with you, but I don't like it." It was at this time that I realized how much my kids were still learning from me. They were still watching, so now I had another decision to make.

Do I teach them to be like Linda friggin Steele and not take shit from anyone? Do I continue to teach them to dig their heels in and DEMAND some goddamn respect? Or do I show them that compromise can be good and doesn't necessarily mean that you're giving in?

I left ZERO room for error. I know this. How could I show them that it is possible to be empathetic and not let somebody walk all over you at the same time when I still was unsure myself? This was a very tough transition for me as I knew it might not only shape my future for a stable relationship, but it could potentially shape my daughters, as well. What happened next was something I had never expected I was capable of doing.

Chapter 35

LEARNING TO BEND

After telling Touchdown I didn't think he was ever going to be capable of understanding my needs, he mentioned a few things he was doing to "work on himself." I was elated because I knew what he had to offer someone. To see him happy would make me happy. Period. Although I was somewhat sad that it would be another woman who would get the best version of him. Still, I was truly happy for him. He was specific with the things he was working on, and it sounded like he had a clear understanding of what it would take to set himself up to be an amazing partner— "regardless of who is at the end of the tunnel"—is exactly what I told him.

Through it all, we were getting closer, finding comfort in each other's words and arms. But I was not going to be fooled again by a man who treated me poorly and then said he would change. Still, I couldn't help but think that this time it looked (and felt) different. For the first time, I met a man who actually went through the steps he needed to in order to make a relationship work. For the first time, I saw actions and not just words … and it got my attention. To me, words without actions backing them up are simply a waste of breath.

Without sharing the personal steps he took to help him grow, I will say that he started actively sharing with me his learnings and findings along the way. He let me in on some valuable insights that made *me* think and tell him out loud, "I am starting to understand a little better that I may not have been perfect either." *Wow, I couldn't just say I was wrong too, could I? No, because I've trained myself to be on the defense my entire life.*

Even though he enlightened me in some respects, I continually reminded him what he needed to change, and that his current behavior wouldn't work for anyone—not me, not anyone. I was relentless. I could never just let up on him. But he didn't back down. He wasn't giving up. He continued to work and show me that he understood. He continued to tell me that he had blind spots and that he is more aware of them now. Rarely during this time did he point the finger at me. And you know his *unresolved past relationships* I mentioned about him earlier? I realized I had them too—of course, I did—and his patience during this time gave me just what I needed to see how *my* behavior affected him. This was a completely new way of thinking for me. I started taking a long hard look within and found that there was no way my past behaviors were going to work for anyone either.

So, we found ourselves in a unique spot. We were in love. But we had created a toxic relationship and pushed each other away in the past because neither of us could recognize our wrongdoings at that time. If we ever wanted to have a long-term companion in our adult lives, we each needed time to fix a few things about ourselves first. Regardless of how this would play out, life is fluid, and I knew that I'd be working daily to build the best version of myself, *for myself*, both mentally and physically. What I started to realize then was I didn't have to be alone to do that, as long as the person I am with is doing the same thing.

I learned a lot about myself during this self-awareness phase. I learned that I suck at trusting men with my feelings. I learned that I suck at forgiving. From my past experiences, forgiving a man meant it was okay for them to do it again, because that's exactly what happened every other time I forgave a man for mistreating me. They would just repeat the same exact behavior. On the flip side, I also learned that if I don't learn to trust, which essentially means vulnerability, the likelihood of me being in any future strong relationship is not good. And I don't want to be alone the rest of my life. I want to share it with someone—with mutual love, trust, and respect.

I have earned the right to have a solid, stable relationship. I have earned the right to have someone treat me with the utmost respect not for all that I have been through, but for finding success despite it all. I have earned the right to feel love, without minimizing the feeling because I am more worried about getting hurt than I am about enjoying my present.

I found someone who is very tolerant and patient and is willing to do whatever it takes to make us work. If I could let my guard down and do the same for him, I could have the companion that I have always wanted. I am learning that I can be vulnerable, but still in control of my life. I truly believe it is possible to have both … and I am living it each day.

I had missed so many things about him. I missed the good things, of course, but I missed my best friend, so I weighed it all out and decided to take this opportunity to teach my daughters, and whoever else was watching (or maybe reading now), how to trust instead of how to dig their heels in and never compromise. *Hahaha, funny, I would be teaching something I knew nothing about—trust.* So, I told myself, *What's the worst that could happen? We break up and I would have to be alone again? Big deal, I've done it before, and I was fine. I can do it again if I have to.* I had nothing to lose and everything to gain, so I gave it a shot. And I am not sorry.

Will we live happily ever after? I hope so! But if we don't, I'm much better equipped on how to move forward with my life on my own terms.

Chapter 36

RESILIENCE AND SUCCESS

What I've come to learn most about myself over my life so far is that regardless of the hand I've been dealt, regardless of how many times I've been knocked down, regardless of the tears I've shed, I get back up each time stronger than before. When relationships end, instead of being mad that I wasted valuable time, I realize that I took the best parts of each one, learned from my experience, and used it to move ahead in life. I realize that each of my experiences taught me something about myself and about life. And that no matter how shitty it can get at times, it is up to me to decide how I want to move forward. Do I want to bury my head in the sand (*so* not my nature) or do I want to stand up and fight. I choose to fight … and I have my entire life.

After every set back, I rebuilt myself. After every time I was pushed down, I found the strength inside me to get back up. I have launched numerous successful businesses, have built an internationally successful brand, and have raised three beautiful, strong daughters. I have rebounded and reinvented myself more times than I can count. While I have always known I was extremely resilient, my life is now my proof.

No one ever told me that I should take negativity and turn it into positivity. But looking back, I was doing that for as long as I can remember. I graduated high school early and catapulted my way to success without looking back. I used all the excruciating and demeaning instances of abuse, not as excuses to fail, but as steppingstones to propel me to the next level. By the time I was 35, I held a top nationally ranked position in my field, and before I turned 43, I built two thriving businesses in different industries, turning my name into an international brand. Every time a man in my life told me I'd fail, I had the attitude of, "Hold my beer, watch this."

If there is one lesson that I hope readers take from this, it's that you are in control of your life … even when you feel like you aren't. No one can take that from you. They can try. And they can make you believe that you don't have any, but ultimately the decision to stay or go, to cry or scream, to give up or move on is your decision, and yours alone. I want you to understand that spotting a pattern is easy once you stop making excuses for that person, stop listening to their justifications for whatever they have done, and stop putting their feelings ahead of your own. Simply, the more chances you give someone, the less they will respect you, and the worse you will feel about yourself.

Trust your instincts and know that you can say goodbye, even if you still love that person. Because if they don't respect you, if they don't honor you, then they don't truly love you the way you deserve. Respect your boundaries and your own self-worth. You will grow from it more than I can explain. You can take every challenge, every obstacle, every setback, every asshole you encounter, and learn something. You will begin to understand that good, bad, or ugly, the experience is preparing you in some way for what is next on your journey.

And I promise you it's not quitting, as the other person will likely try to make you think—or maybe some small voice inside you is whispering in your ear. Make no mistake that walking away from a toxic situation is *not quitting*—it is not giving up—it is survival. We will never succeed in a relationship, in business, or in life if we stay in a situation that no longer serves us or is blatantly harmful to us because we don't want to be a quitter. Being successful means knowing when to pivot. And that is what this is about—switching lanes to a path of being fulfilled, being successful, and being happy.

Once you remove yourself from those situations, you'll have more time and energy to spend on those who bring you up, not push you down. You'll have more time to do what you love, without fear or anxiety, without doubt or worry. Make a commitment to yourself to put everything you have into what fuels you from this day forward and watch the transformation. Trust me, it happens. Those who knew me at the beginning of writing this book saw me evolve right before their very eyes. It's just what happens when you make the decision to put yourself first.

Both in training and in life, I promise you, the more you put into it, the more you'll get out of it.

EPILOGUE

The funny thing about life is that even when we think we have figured it all out, even when we think we've overcome our last obstacle, even when we think we have learned everything there is to learn, we're shown that even the most fundamental things we think we know for sure, we don't know at all …

5/1/19

Dear Mr. Cerone,

My name is Linda Steele. A few months ago, I decided to do the Ancestry DNA test that my daughter had bought me for Christmas. I saw you signed on after my results came in, so my name may look familiar. You probably saw my daughter's name and my name just a few down the list from yours. I am going to cut right to the chase … I am your half-sister.

When my results came back, I took a screenshot of the names on the list to show my mom and my daughters how I didn't recognize the other name that kept coming up on my list (Cerone). I had been searching for my dad's sibling's names. But there was one person who recognized the name Cerone, and that was my mom.

So, after the shock wore off, she called me and asked me to come over because she had something she had to tell me in person. After 48 years of her not being 100% sure whose child I was, it was confirmed, before her very own eyes.

I am hoping you'd like to hear the story and that you will contact me. I will understand if it takes you a little bit to process this news. It took me two months to write this letter. I promised my daughters I would wait thirty days to do anything. Then it took me another thirty days to get up the nerve.

I am not trying to disrupt your family. I have a family too, so I understand. I am simply hoping that you will be as curious as I am and that you are open to discuss this situation. ☺

Sincerely,
Linda Steele

And so, a new chapter begins …

My mother always taught me,
"Unless you've walked a mile in my stilettos,
do not judge me."

So, I don't.

ABOUT THE AUTHOR

First-time author Linda Steele is a creative, passionate and dedicated entrepreneur determined to improve the lives of others through safe, efficient fitness. As a certified personal trainer, a performance nutrition and exercise therapy specialist, a podcast and radio show co-host, and a professional model, she believes that small goals and lifestyle changes can grow into massive accomplishments. Linda has successfully been helping clients reach their health and fitness goals for over eighteen years by putting their bodies in a state where they are no longer dependent on blood pressure meds, cholesterol meds or anti-depressants. She has spent most of her career training clients to care for their bodies by helping them better understand the body-mind connection. Her three-prong fitness, nutrition, and well-being approach have transformed countless lives.

To Learn More About Linda:

LindaSteeleWellness.com

https://nervesofsteele.net/program/

NervesofSteele.net

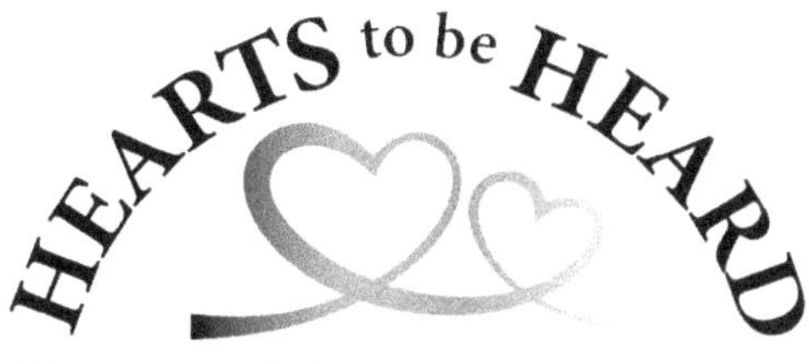

With every donation, a voice will be given to
the creativity that lies within the hearts of
our children living with diverse challenges.

By making this difference, children that may
not have been given the opportunity to have their
Heart Heard will have the freedom to create
beautiful works of art and musical creations.

Donate by visiting

HeartstobeHeard.com

We thank you.

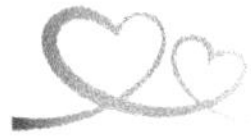

www.ingramcontent.com/pod-product-compliance
Lightning Source LLC
Chambersburg PA
CBHW051759050726
47598CB00006B/2351